About the author

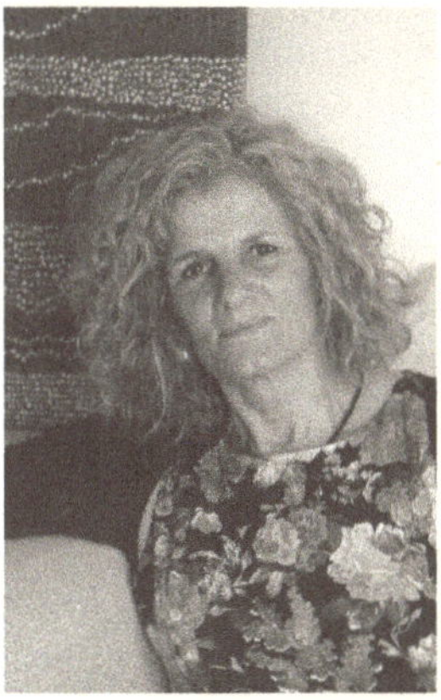

Rhea Dempsey is a highly sought after childbirth educator, speaker, counsellor and birth attendant with experience at over one thousand births. She is respected as one of Australia's foremost thinkers on the topic of working with pain in childbirth and its connection to normal physiological birthing. With three adult daughters of her own, Rhea's understanding of birth has been gained during thirty-seven years working with pregnant women, their partners, support people, midwives and medical practitioners.

Praise for *Birth with Confidence*

Over many years I have observed Rhea Dempsey's wisdom and brilliance in working with birthing women; I am so glad she has finally written this book. Your birth experience can colour your mothering from the beginning.

It can leave you feeling strong—a confident woman who trusts her body and herself as a mother—or it can leave you fragile and doubting your ability to nurture.

Rhea is number one at preparing women for a powerful birthing experience that will set them up to start their mothering journey with strength and confidence. If you are pregnant or considering getting pregnant, this book is a must-read!

Pinky McKay, parenting and lactation expert, author of *Parenting by Heart, Toddler Tactics, 100 Ways to Calm the Crying* and *Sleeping Like a Baby*

Rhea's book is the book I wish I'd had before my first baby—it puts words to the gut feelings I have about birth. This book is a game-changer for us women who are neither hippies nor radicals, but simply wish to have a go at normal birth because we know there is a more richly rewarding way for both mothers and babies.

Leigh Russell, TV presenter, sports management consultant, leadership coach

During my twenty years of involvement in childbirth activism and research, many women have asked me 'How can I have a good birth?' I have wanted just this book—Rhea's wise answers—to give them. Now we have it.

Dr Kerreen Reiger, School of Social Sciences, La Trobe University and author of *Our Bodies Our Babies: The forgotten women's movement*

Just finished reading *Birth with Confidence: Savvy choices for normal birth* by Rhea Dempsey. Fantastic book! It really encourages women to explore and reflect on what they want and provides guidance about how to navigate the 'maternity system' and the birthing process. This is the information mothers need … holistic and woman-centered rather than the usual manuals on the 'stages' of labour and how to be a good girl in hospital.

Rachel Reed, PhD, midwife, lecturer

Rhea Dempsey's dedication to educating and empowering women to achieve the natural birth they desire has been a shining light on the Australian birthing scene for almost three decades. What a gift to finally have her unique wisdom and boundless passion on the pages of a book from which many more women and families can benefit.

Jo Askham and Jess Permezel, past national convenors of Choices for Childbirth

Using Rhea's wealth of knowledge and understanding about women, their bodies and their perceptions of themselves in labour, this book takes a unique look at the power of working with pain and the amazing things a woman can do as a result of it. Rather than the traditional labour and birth book about what to expect, this book is ideal for those women who wish to know how to work with their labour and what strategies to put in place to help them achieve the best possible outcome for them and their baby.

Melinda Eales, midwife, childbirth education specialist, trainer

Rhea Dempsey has been nourishing women of childbearing age and the Childbirth Education community for more than thirty years. An inspirational speaker, a natural facilitator of groups, and a birth attendant of extraordinary ability, Rhea is 'une sage femme'—the French term for midwife that, literally translated, is 'a wise woman'. I will be wholeheartedly recommending Rhea's book to women who plan to have a child, women who have had a traumatic birth and want something better and new midwives, so that they may better understand the wonder of birth.

Christine Powell, registered nurse, midwife, lactation consultant and maternal and child health nurse

In supporting women and in experiencing Rhea's training ourselves, we have seen the lights go on for couples who suddenly understand the ancient wisdom of their bodies and the psychological factors at work that can enliven or inhibit their birth experience. This understanding and knowing how to work with it has been transformational not only to birth experiences but to the relationship of many couples we have worked with. We are thrilled that *Birth with Confidence* has finally arrived, making available Rhea's extensive experience and profound perspective on birth in what she aptly calls the 'labour-bypass era'. With normal birth under threat from a culture of fear and medicalisation, this work is an inspiring investigation of the complex psychological, physical and societal pressures coming to bear on a process we have been successfully experiencing for eons: birth! Rhea's capacity to shed light on these factors is unique, insightful and transformative.

Milly Dabrowski and Charmaine Dennis, directors of Fertile Ground Health Group, Melbourne, Australia

Ever since I encountered first-hand the power and the clarity of Rhea Dempsey's vision of childbirth, I have been hoping Rhea would write a book. Now, having synthesised and distilled more than thirty years of experience, observation and analysis, Rhea's book goes straight to the heart of the matter. Her voice is unmistakable—forceful, lucid and startlingly eloquent. She is never didactic or preachy. Her every word oozes honesty and a profound respect for women. Rhea Dempsey is, in other words, the real deal: one of this country's most formidable minds on the subject of childbirth. I have no doubt her book will become an instant classic—for women about to give birth, for their partners, and for childbirth professionals across Australia and beyond.

Maria Tumarkin, author of *Otherland*, *Traumascapes* and *Courage*

Praise for the author

Rhea Dempsey is a wise woman who everyone I know refers to everyone else I know, all the time. She is a keeper of secrets and a polisher of treasures. She is a fierce supporter of things that actually matter: like women and their experience when giving birth, and men and their experience of bonding with their children. These are just two of the things that make her a true treasure, and we are so lucky she's written some of her wisdom down in this book.

Clare Bowditch, musician, entrepreneur

Through her wisdom and skill, Rhea helps couples recognise the multi-dimensional nature of birth and encourages them to use the experience as an opportunity for profound personal growth.

Professor Marc Cohen, foundation head, Department of Complementary Medicine, Royal Melbourne Institute of Technology

My clients who work with Rhea are better prepared for the challenges of labour. And those who have her attend their births get to experience her unique presence. Rhea's wisdom and intuition, derived from decades of support, provide tools to empower, resulting in a satisfying birth experience.

Jennie Teskey, independent midwife and counsellor

Rhea tells it like it is. Best birth education money can buy.

Annie Sprague, independent midwife, maternal and child health nurse, and author of *Water Labour Water Birth*

Rhea has an un-romanticised belief that ordinary people can do extraordinary things. When she walks into a room and starts talking or accompanies you through a forty-hour labour, it seems everyone else starts to believe the same thing.

Emily Lubitz (Tin Pan Orange) and Harry Angus (The Cat Empire), musicians

Rhea Dempsey is a loved and admired birth educator. While researching for our documentaries, we were seeking the expertise of the world's top natural birth practitioners. Rhea's name kept coming up, due to her vast experience and the stories of recommendation and gratitude from many, many women and families whom she suppported during birth and postpartum. We sought Rhea out, I attended many workshops and conducted in-depth interviews, part of which became a vital part of our films *The Face of Birth* and *Meet the Experts*. I would recommend her services to any expecting parents.

Kate Gorman, co writer/director/producer of *The Face of Birth*

Rhea Dempsey is a national treasure. Her wisdom and experience around the process of natural birthing is a gift to all women who wish to enter their birthing journey with a sense of empowerment and intention. Birth is a huge event in any woman's life and rarely is the space provided for such deeply thoughtful preparation as Rhea provides in her workshops. I feel blessed to have been able to give birth naturally to my two children, in large part nourished by an understanding that pain can be power. I hope with all my heart that there is a Rhea Dempsey of the future to look after my daughter and all women who wish to embrace their power and bring their children into the world with consciousness.

Berry Liberman, publisher and editor of *Dumbo Feather*

Rhea gave me a priceless gift going into my birth—a sense of self-belief. My husband and I felt confident and capable throughout the entire labour. Rhea's warmth, insight, pragmatism and sense of humour sets her apart as a birth educator. The knowledge Rhea equipped my husband and I with ultimately made the birth of our son a truly wondrous experience. It set us up perfectly for a happy home and a happy baby and as a result we will forever treasure the birth of our first child.

Sophie Black, former editor of *Crikey*

Birth *with* Confidence

Savvy choices for normal birth

RHEA DEMPSEY

BOAT
HOUSE
PRESS

Published by Boathouse Press
Box 405 Fairfield 3078

First published in 2013 by Boathouse Press
Reprinted 2014, 2017

Cover design by Sandra Nobes
Text design and typesetting by Megan Ellis
Printed in Australia by Griffin Press

National Library of Australia Cataloguing-in-Publication entry

Author:	Dempsey, Rhea.
Title:	Birth with confidence: savvy choices for normal birth / Rhea Dempsey.
ISBN:	9780987402905 (pbk.)
Subjects:	Childbirth. Labor (Obstetrics) Pregnancy. Health.
Dewey Number:	618.2

For Polly, who first planted the seed

Author's note

While many of the names of women, partners, babies, midwives and birth attendants used in the many stories told in this book are actual names, some have been changed for reasons of privacy.

My usual reference to 'her' when talking about a baby can be explained by my having birthed three daughters.

Finally, while this book is intended to support women to undertake normal physiological birth, it is by no means meant to convey that normal birth is possible in every circumstance. Regardless of a woman's or caregiver's intentions, there will be some birth situations that require the best that modern medicine has to offer in order to keep mothers and babies safe.

Contents

Introduction

The birth of my first daughter was a version of the standard hospital birth of the time—augmentation (use of synthetic hormones to speed up the labour), pethidine (narcotic drug), episiotomy (incision to the perineum), and emergency manual removal of the placenta after the cord broke during a forcefully managed third stage. Finally came the routine separation from my baby for six hours after she was born.

It was not what I expected. I was devastated. Over the two days I spent in hospital after her birth I felt I was quietly going crazy, until finally, in despair, I found myself crying in the toilet, full of conflicting feelings I didn't yet understand. Then, forty-eight hours after my daughter's birth, supported by my husband and mother—and guided by instincts and longings that were at odds with hospital routines and directives—I discharged myself and my baby from hospital against 'expert' advice.

In taking my daughter home that day, I was acting from deep protective instincts that had awakened in me in those two days after her birth. Gradually, all my senses had come alive to her. I became captivated by her smell, delighted by the softness of her skin and feel of her body, by her sounds and her taste as I smooched and nibbled at her fingers and toes. I was loving and bonding with her as I gazed endlessly into her eyes. My mothering hormones, and the instinctive longings flowing from them, emerged.

Taking her home at that time marked a transformation in me and became one of the most profound decisions of my life. This was the moment I was born as a mother.

In the years since, I have realised that this transformational moment—this connection with my feelings and instincts—need not have waited until days after the birth. It need not have taken two days of despair. In fact, I could have been connected with these deeper, transformational instincts during the birth itself. Instead, my birth experience had eroded my trust in my feelings and my connection with my baby. It was this that saddened me in the aftermath of my first birthing experience; the sense of a lost opportunity. I asked myself, 'How did it happen?'

I had come to the birth of this first daughter with a trust and belief in myself based on years of physical pursuits and challenging experiences. I was a fit, healthy, independent, resourceful young woman in a committed relationship, ready to have a much-wanted baby. I was a physical education teacher, a swimming and outdoor adventure instructor, an adventurous traveller, a feminist and a self-determining woman. I trusted my body; it had always served me well. And I believed pregnancy, birth and breastfeeding would again be body experiences that would confirm this trust.

I believed birthing was a normal function of a healthy body, not an illness, and that my body would just know what to do. And I believed—naïvely, I realised later—that the birth culture, with its experts, practices and procedures, was set up to support and facilitate *my* capacity to give birth, not (as proved to be the case), to control and undermine it.

In hindsight, I can see that the loss of this strong trust in my body and my instincts happened subtly. The slippage started during the pregnancy, under the barrage of routine medical tests that, even while confirming I was low risk, nonetheless caused me to feel that perhaps I couldn't trust my body. After all, my medical caregivers appeared very worried about it. They insisted on doing this, watching that—all because pregnancy and birth were apparently so very unpredictable and dangerous. So I began to believe this myself. They were the experts after all; they must know, mustn't they? Gradually, as my pregnancy progressed, I gave my trust away and with it my personal agency. My power.

So my first regret was the way I let my medical carers erode the years of trust I had built in my own body. The second—again, as a result of the 'conditioned' trust placed in my carers and the medical system—was that I didn't follow my instincts about the location of the birth.

At the time of my first pregnancy, I was living in England and had friends who had had homebirths. This option felt right to me, though I didn't really know then what it was that I was responding to in myself, in trying to organise a homebirth. But I was thwarted in these attempts because the protocols for homebirth in the UK at the time meant that only second and subsequent babies could be born at home. So I was dissuaded from following my feelings. Instead of the homebirth I was drawn to, I fell into acquiescence—which is how I eventually ended up in a large teaching hospital in north London, a million miles from my feelings.

My third regret was for my naïve acquiescence during the birth itself.

On the day of my daughter's birth I was hardly aware I was in labour. My mother had arrived from Australia that morning and we spent the day catching up and opening endless cards and baby presents from my extended family back home. This was a delightful distraction so it wasn't until late in the evening that the slow leak of my waters made sense of the discomforts I had been feeling throughout the day. I was beginning to labour.

After phoning the hospital to let them know my waters were leaking, the response, without explanation, was to send an ambulance to bring me to hospital immediately. This set off a deep anxiety in me. Did this dramatic response mean that something was going wrong?

At the hospital, everybody, including me, was surprised to find, on vaginal examination, that I was already well into the first stage of labour at 6 cm dilated, and everything was fine. From this point on, however, the labour—which had obviously been progressing smoothly with very little demand on me—stopped completely.

Over the next seven hours a standoff developed between my husband and me on the one hand, and the medical staff on the other. Although the baby and I were well, the hospital staff wanted to put up a drip of synthetic hormones to get the labour going again, in accordance with the hospital's routine medical protocol. Still trusting my body, I wanted to let it get back into its own rhythm.

Gradually though, we became worn down by the hourly battles with the staff, which ended in me being trundled off on a trolley and left in the small ante-room leading to the pan room. Eventually, inevitably, we acquiesced, and the drip was started, followed by an unannounced and unrequested routine shot of pethidine (my baby was still suffering from the effect of this drug on her breathing when she was born). Then came the stirrups, a routine episiotomy, an emergency manual removal of the placenta after the umbilical cord broke during an aggressively managed third stage, and the routine separation from my baby for the first six hours after she was born. This hurtling 'cascade of interventions' (not that I was familiar with this term at the time) left my husband and me, not to mention our baby, in a state of shock. *What the fuck had just happened?*

During pregnancy I had done some research into the hospital's routine practices and asked what I had thought were the right questions. I remember asking, at an information session conducted at the hospital, what their policy was on routine episiotomies and being reassured that they only performed them if medically necessary. Now, during my birth, and with no explanations given, I was subjected to an episiotomy.

In my short time in the large communal post-natal ward, a radicalisation process began. I discovered that of the twelve women on the ward, ten had had episiotomies, while the other two had had caesarean deliveries. So in this birthplace they obviously believed all women needed episiotomies! This speaks volumes. It speaks of a belief that women's bodies are not well designed for birthing—and the influence of this belief on medical practice. And so another veil was lifted and my third regret revealed—regret at my naïve acquiescence to the authority of this maternity institution.

I understand now, after years of experience and with an awareness of the influence of fear and adrenalin on birth, that my labour could have unfolded differently—straightforwardly, as I had intended. If, when my labour stalled at 6 cm, I had received support to move, to walk, to express my fears and to trust myself, instead of being pressured and badgered, I would have found a way back into my labour.

Or if, in fact, I'd just been encouraged to return home, or to stay at home in the first place, until my labour was fully established; or if I'd known then that different care settings can have different routine protocols—then things could have gone differently.

What I didn't consciously understand at the time but rather felt intuitively, was the importance of 'feelings'—the importance of both the feeling of safe, familiar territory and the feeling of emotional safety, which leads to physiological soothing or 'felt security' as it is sometimes called. Both of these feelings have been confirmed by research in recent years to have great impact on our hormones and therefore on our birthing capacity. If only I had known this consciously at the time.

In trying to understand what took place during this labour and how I came to be so separated from my feelings and consequently from my body and my baby, I have had to reflect on the influence that the medical systems entrusted with my care had on me. I now see that, like so many first-time mothers, I was unconsciously acting out of what we can call 'the trance of acquiescence'—the culturally conditioned trance activated when faced with medical authority.

In the hospital after my first birth, the continuing routine separation of my baby and me (in what I had been told during pregnancy was a 'rooming-in' hospital) only allowed us short times together during her four-hourly feeds. But this was enough time for her to weave her captivating magic. I wanted to keep her snuggled close to me, rather than putting her back in the nursery—and yet putting her back there is what I was being instructed to do.

Over that first forty-eight hours, the gap between my instinctive feelings (what I yearned to do) and my culturally patterned response to medical authority (acquiescing to what others expected and instructed me to do) grew wider and wider, leading to that life-changing decision to take her home.

This was my birthing experience: so different from what I had expected. It affected me deeply. So what? you may ask. After all, I had a healthy baby. Does it matter how the birth itself unfolded?

In the years since, I have come to realise that for many, many women, it does matter. I listen again and again to women in debriefing sessions (or a workshop or pregnancy class, or coffee shop, or supermarket or party), as they talk about their distress about birth experiences that have unfolded so differently to their expectations and potential.

Yes, they have a healthy baby, a 'good' outcome—if we look only through the narrow frame of medical criteria. Yet if we widen our frame to include a view of the overall wellbeing of the mother and baby, we might question this 'good' outcome and our present birth culture's means of achieving it.

With a baby in her arms but with her sense of self shattered, a mother asks herself, 'What happened?'—just as I asked myself after the birth of my first daughter.

Like me, they wonder where things went wrong. Like me, they went into their birthing experience thinking: 'birthing is a normal healthy process; the choices I'm making seem to be what's expected and supported and what most women are making, so this must be what normal birth takes. This must be what I should trust.'

And why shouldn't they trust? Why shouldn't any new mother trust? Why shouldn't I, a new mother facing the unknown, have trusted thirty-five years ago? Who else would we trust but the caregivers and maternity system sanctioned by our culture to care for our transition into motherhood and our baby's coming into the world?

For me, the sadness of my first daughter's birth was my lack of awareness of what could help my birthing capacity. This sadness was further compounded when I realised that the people I had entrusted with our care did not understand what helped the normal physical process of birth to unfold either—they, too, had lost touch with this knowledge. We were all struggling under the weight of this loss.

In the countless births I have attended over the past thirty-odd years, I have come to see that the real story and potential for any birth is revealed when we understand the holistic nature of the experience. A mother's birthing capacity is affected by her culture's values and attitudes, her own values and attitudes, her life experiences, and her trust in, and lived experience of, her body. This includes her experience of her sexuality, her own experience of being born, her experience of being mothered and her generational birthing patterns. A woman's birthing capacity is affected by her relationship with her partner, her fears, her readiness for her baby and her willingness (or not) to engage with the challenging embodiment of birthing—pain.

Facing pain in labour is undoubtedly an even greater challenge for contemporary women birthing in an environment where the seduction of the epidural is everywhere lauded. For me, pain was not the overwhelming issue. My years of physical activity had accustomed me to being well outside my comfort zone while working through pain zones. The issue for me was a lack of any holistic understanding.

This was the knowledge I wish a wise birthing woman had bequeathed to me before my first daughter's birth. I now understand that the story of her birth could have unfolded without the need for medical intervention. It could have confirmed my competent sense of self, strengthened my capacity for mothering and facilitated my bonding with my baby. When my labour stalled, I needed a trusted caregiver filled with age-old birthing wisdom, offering patience, encouragement and guidance to support me back into my birthing rhythm.

In study after study around the world, we have come to see that normal physiological birthing is best supported when birthing women are accompanied by caregivers who are experienced in normal physiological childbirth, known to them through pregnancy, and with them one on one and continuously throughout the labour. This is what's needed for normal birth.

I didn't know at my first labour, what I have since realised—that in order to give myself a chance of birthing normally, I needed to be very proactive in protecting my birthing potential. I needed to have researched actual statistics in that hospital rather than being lulled by the general answers to my questions. I needed to see if their 'walk' matched their 'talk' in order to have made wise choices to back my birthing potential and to match my trust and beliefs about birth.

What saddens me now is that, in the current birth climate, the conditions needed to enable women to birth in harmony with their instincts, intentions and potential are even less available than they were to me back then. A woman wishing for a normal birth, the way I had wished for one, would find it even harder today.

As well as the delight of my daughter herself, the extra gift of her birth was my becoming aware of a holistic understanding of birth. It led me, initially, into the work of supporting mothers and babies in the ways I wish I had been supported when I had my first child. I started attending births and then trained as a childbirth educator and began facilitating workshops, seminars and training courses. Finally I trained as a counsellor in order to offer counselling to pregnant women, new mothers and couples.

It was also this new knowledge and awakening that helped me when, two years after the birth of our first baby and back in Australia, our second beautiful daughter arrived. This pregnancy, labour and birth were an affirmation and celebration of the journey that had been started by my first daughter's birth. My feelings were strong and clear. I followed them confidently and I connected with people who validated my 'knowing'. A homebirth this time was the obvious consequence of all the knowledge I had gained and the changes I had made within myself.

What a wonderful time we had on that Saturday thirty-three years ago when she came to be with us. A great welcoming party, her father, her 'big' sister, support people, birth attendant and doctor—ten of us there in a loving circle to welcome her. I was never separated from my instincts or feelings and so bonded with her immediately.

Birthing was still challenging but with it came such a feeling of celebration and support. In early second stage, as my daughter was beginning to move down, but before the outrageous sensations of 'crowning' had pulled me back into my body, I remember being in a timeless, expansive place, feeling myself open to all the energies of the universe rushing through me and manifesting as the most glorious singing.

I sang out this birth song again some two years later on a work-a-day Wednesday morning when our third darling daughter made her way into the world. A peaceful feeling of family life unfolded, during another beautiful homebirth, another experience of surrender and another experience of transcendence. Her father, her two 'big' sisters and her aunty were present, with the doctor making it just in time.

This song was old, instinctive—archetypal. I felt connected to all birthing women, back through time, into the future and in the present. The song came from a surrender to the power of my birthing instincts.

I've since heard this ancient song hundreds of times—the birth song, with its echoes of a universal experience, overlaid by each woman's personal musical tone and signature.

My work in birth feels like an exploration to regain lost wisdom, wisdom that may increase the possibility of normal, spontaneous birthing. My awareness of this birthing wisdom has been opened to me through the births of my daughters and through the blessing of being with mothers and babies and their families at over 1000 births. And it has come from what I have learned from interactions with women and their partners in my classes, workshops, seminars and counselling work.

I've also absorbed knowledge and wisdom from the many midwives, childbirth educators and birth activists with whom I've been thankful to work. So, in this book, the voices, knowledge and spirit of many others will be present. Not least, I am drawing on the instinctive teachings that have emerged from within the birthing women themselves and from the whisperings of all those sweet new babes, filled with such knowing as they enter our arms.

Women who have a yearning for normal birth today face all the obstacles I faced at my first daughter's birth, and more. They cannot afford to be naïve, the way I was. They need to be willing to undertake the challenges of birth, but more than that, they need knowledge about what will help them reach their full birthing potential.

Helping women gain this knowledge and to make wise choices, savvy choices, to support their potential for normal birth is the purpose of this book.

1

The birth you want: what motivates the willing woman?

What do I need to know about birth, Rhea? This is a question I've been asked and been answering for the past thirty-five years. My response has changed radically over that time.

I used to answer by talking about contractions, breathing, stages of labour … all that body stuff. These days, before I answer the question, I ask my own question—what type of birth are you hoping for? It's a given, of course, that every woman wants what we all want, a healthy mother and baby. What I'm asking is how do they want to go about that? Being clear about this at the outset is important because what a pregnant woman needs to know about birth is quite different depending on her answer to this question.

Do they want to be an active participant in the birth? Do they want their baby to be an active participant in its own birth? Or do they want their caregivers to be the active agents who take over the work of delivering the baby? Basically, do they want to put in, do they want to work with their bodies and babies—do they have any yearning for normal physiological birth?

What exactly do I mean by normal physiological birth? Let me explain. I am talking about a birth that is initiated by the hormonal interplay stimulated by the baby's readiness to be born and the mother's readiness to release her. This is a birth where the labour is driven by surging birth hormones, hormones that drive the intensifying contractions—longer, stronger, closer-together contractions that open your body. Hormones that stimulate 'bearing down' urges to bring your baby onto your perineum, setting off a further surge of hormones that peak with an 'oxytocin high' at the moments of birth—a multi-tasking 'love bombing' that awakens your bonding behaviours, attunes your senses towards your exquisite new baby, and stimulates breastfeeding. Hormones that, at the same time, initiate the passing of the placenta and the contracting of the uterus to mark the completion of the birth.

If a woman tells me she wants this kind of birth, she is what I call a 'willing woman': willing to engage with the birth process, willing to engage with her body, her feelings, her fears. Willing to engage with the challenge.

One of the most popular workshops I run is called Embracing the Intensity: transforming pain in labour. With a title like that I think it's safe to say I draw the 'willing' crowd.

In this workshop, I ask women, their partners and support people to reflect on why normal physiological birth is important to them. I ask them this because normal physiological birth is a hard gig that is no longer valued at a societal level. I know these women need to be very clear about their own reasons for having a go at it.

Here are some of the responses they give to this question:

Instead of lying down I want to use all the active birth positions. That makes sense to me and I know it will give the baby the best opportunity for a good birth—Jane

I want to optimise the health of my baby, to make use of my body's ability to birth my baby and have a speedier recovery after the birth—Kathy

I want my baby to be fully present and not 'drugged out' when he/she arrives and I want to feel my body working, feel the pain of birthing—Sandra

I want to stay in touch with what's going on. None of the pain-relief options seem to come without a price—nausea, loss of mobility, etc. I want to be able to do this myself and avoid the two caesareans my mother had—Tracy

I feel in my last two births the pain relief (gas, pethidine, epidural) didn't help; in fact it created other problems, especially the epidural, which, at least in part, resulted in me having a caesarean—Susie

We conceived this baby, now I want to work actively with my partner, working together to birth our baby, not have somebody else take it over—Patricia

Health and wellbeing

One of the most common motivations for a woman who wants to undertake normal physiological childbirth is her understanding of the benefits for her baby's wellbeing. She understands that, in the main, pregnancy, labour and birth are 'wellness' states, so she wants to optimise the normal physiological process.

During pregnancy she has probably attended to her health by focusing on her nutrition, her activity levels, her sleep and rest cycles, her relaxation and stress balance, and by changing behaviours that have not been compatible with her own or her baby's health and wellbeing. She has stopped doing this and eating that, she has taken all the best advice to maximise her baby's growth and development.

So she does not want to erode the results of all that diligence during the birth itself by being pumped with synthetic hormones, drugs or routine antibiotics that pass through to her baby as well as compromising her own health. Nor does she want her baby to be poked, prodded, scraped, jabbed, pulled, twisted, separated or taken away from her and isolated after the birth.

If she's done some research, she may have an understanding that in normal physiological birth she is going to maximise the possibility of the baby receiving protective bacteria from her as it passes through her vagina, consequently minimising the baby's vulnerability to asthma, allergies and infection. She is thinking of the benefits—for the baby's alertness and adjustment to life outside the womb—of a birth that means it is not 'zonked out' on drugs, or needing to clear synthetic hormones, drugs or 'just in case' antibiotics from its system. And she may also know about the figures that suggest babies born by elective caesarean are three times more likely to need neo-natal intensive care. She wants the baby to be able to use its instincts to assist the birth process and be primed for bonding and breastfeeding.

Some women are aware, too, of the connection between easier and earlier establishment of breastfeeding and normal physiological birth. This connection is due to the woman and baby being undisturbed in the critical period immediately after birth. Primed by their hormones during this crucial first hour, the mother's and baby's instincts for breastfeeding are activated and in sync. In contrast to the babies born through a normal physiological birth process—who are more likely to be immediately placed in their mother's arms—babies delivered by the use of forceps or vacuum extraction, or by caesarean, may be separated from the mother for various medical checks, which can mean a delay or disturbance in the early breastfeeding connection.

Some of those who attend my workshops are aware that they are more likely to have a speedier physical recovery from a birth that has not involved synthetic hormones and drugs of one type or another, which need to be cleared from their system; and has not included the use of forceps, vacuum extraction or episiotomy, which usually result in bruising, stitches and discomfort. Of course, they are also onto the fact that they will have a speedier recovery from a normal physiological birth than they will from the major abdominal surgery involved in a caesarean.

Finally, many of the women in my workshops and classes will be keen to have a go at normal physiological birth because they have an understanding of the hormones that are released through this process. These are hormones that not only drive the contractions, but also prime the mother and the baby for that 'love rush' at birth, and for the laying down of the earliest physiological foundations for a secure attachment that will support the baby's ongoing physical and emotional wellbeing.

They might also understand that normal physiological labour and birth, because of the need it creates for intense physical and emotional support, means they will be working closely with their partner and other support people, sweating and straining together, making eye contact and breathing together, massaging and bonding together. All of this means that everyone gets a dose of those love hormones and so are *all* primed for the love rush when the baby is born.

Now, I have been present at births where epidurals have become necessary and I have to say there is a difference in the 'welcoming' energy, 'the vibe'... call it what you will! This is so, even when the whole support team is working to keep a loving focus by consciously attuning to the mother and baby. It's the absence of all the natural oxytocin and endorphins swirling around—the joint just ain't jumping in the same way!

The willing women attending my classes have some understanding of the fact that, unless it's absolutely medically necessary, *nobody* should miss out on the hormonal multiplier effect that normal physiological birth offers and the 'love bombing' that results—especially not that new baby.

A path to transformation

Many women who come to my workshops also feel that undertaking the challenge of a normal physiological birth offers a capacity-building opportunity, an opportunity to develop their inner strength and boost their personal and inter-personal resource base.

These women are viewing birth from what we might call a 'growth perspective' or 'capacity building' mindset. They might be placing birth in the context of challenging life experiences that demand, as birthing woman Jules said, 'all those resources of determination, of courage, of endurance'—all those character markers.

A 'growth mindset' provides motivation for engaging with painful challenging processes, whether they relate to extending physical skill and endurance, confronting fears, developing understanding, enhancing emotional intelligence, increasing resilience or spiritual growth.

A growth mindset—actively taking on experiences that expand our mental, emotional, physical or psychological comfort zones—is valued, espoused and glorified in many areas of life but not, it seems, in birthing. In fact, when it comes to birth, we'd have to say that instead a pitying, 'Oh, you poor thing', *diminishment* mindset seems to prevail. Willing women in my workshops aren't buying into this, they are keen to apply a growth mindset to their birth experience.

The desire of many women to experience normal physiological birth may be driven by factors they can't necessarily articulate, but which can perhaps be understood with the help of some psychological theories.

Women instinctively drawn to the idea of a normal physiological birth might come at it from an innate sense of valuing expansive and growth-filled ways of being in life—what the field of Positive Psychology[1] (which is concerned with our strengths, fulfilment and what makes life most worth living) would suggest is the pursuit of 'flourishing'[2] in life.

New mother Sue demonstrates this perspective when she describes her birth experience as 'something that's set me on an entirely new path. It's a birth for me as well because I've allowed those strengths to really flow through to other areas of my life, I've allowed myself to experience this in a way that I haven't let myself experience a lot of other life-affirming events. It's absolutely transformational'.

Coming under the umbrella of Positive Psychology, two other emerging psychological theories—'flow' and 'hope'—also provide support for the willing woman's desire for normal physiological birth.

Normal physiological birth is a perfect vehicle for experiencing what's called a 'flow' state. Whether they call it that or not, people everywhere are hunting down flow experiences—in their creative expression, their study, productive work, hobbies, physical achievements, meditation, and relaxation ... the list goes on.

Flow happens when experience seamlessly unfolds moment to moment and we enter a state of intense and focused concentration on the present moment. We lose self-consciousness, time passes faster than normal, and we gain an innate sense of how to respond to whatever comes next. Journalist Amanda Hooton referred to this in a recent article about Olympic athletes.[3] It's a 'mysterious mental blessing' she says.

Normal physiological birth has absolutely got flow covered. Undisturbed and well-supported willing birthing women who are guided by their hormonally triggered instincts and unafraid to work strongly with their bodies, enter a deep flow state. Research into flow confirms that when this state is achieved it is intrinsically rewarding, life affirming and growth filled—what a pay-off for the birthing mum and her baby!

'Hope theory' is based on understanding that much of human behaviour is goal-directed. These goals can be conscious or unconscious and can be either 'approach' or 'avoidance' goals. Whether we feel hopeful enough to take on approach goals (developmental, growth-filled, challenging, learning goals) or whether, instead, we put our available energy into avoidance goals (all manner of behaviours, diversions and procrastinations whose primary aim is to protect us from the distress of possible failure, rejection, judgement and shame), basically comes down to whether we have been supported enough in life to feel hopeful and capable. Or whether the lack of (or type of) support we have received in our life has led to repeated experiences of feeling hopeless and incapable.

There can be confusion though about what can be considered approach goals and avoidance goals when it comes to birthing. This is because, whatever a woman's personal life experiences are in relation to feelings of 'hopefulness' or 'hopelessness', contemporary birthing women in general are so bombarded with negative birth stories, they are bound to hold some feelings of hopelessness in regard to birthing.

So there is a complexity that can blur the motivations of the contemporary birthing woman. What will constitute an approach goal or an avoidance goal for an individual birthing woman? Is she motivated to 'approach' the experience of working with her body? Or is she motivated to 'approach' controlling and numbing her birthing body?

I'm assuming that a willing woman will, at least in theory, be motivated to approach working with her body, but the dominant cultural messages and biases about birth are also alive in her psyche and can erupt to undermine her conscious intentions—especially when the labour builds and the going gets tough.

Positive Psychology, and flow and hope theories haven't addressed birthing specifically, but we could imagine that if they did, they would suggest that birth experiences that offer women opportunities to build resilience—to have an increased sense of their personal resources and strengths following the birth experience—would be preferred as a foundation for mothering.

Related to these psychological understandings is the perspective of those willing women who choose to engage with birthing as a 'rite of passage'. Some women treat it as a test of courage, a pathway to strengthen their inner resources for mothering. They take it on as a modern-day heroine's journey—a quest to overcome obstacles and confront themselves.

Says Nancy:

> I've got an interest in knowing myself better, deeper—and I knew that birthing had the potential of giving that to me. It was an opportunity I didn't want to pass up. I wanted the best opportunity possible. It's a rite of passage. I was going to get a real insight into myself, which is something I wanted.

Some, like Jules, feel the benefits of this rite of passage will also be conferred to her baby:

> I felt, in terms of the baby, I actually wanted her to be born into all those resources of determination, of courage, of endurance and all those resources you need to have in order to give birth naturally. She was exposed to them in her birth. I wanted those qualities to be present for her when she arrived.

Some women frame the birth experience as 'soul work'. They understand that pain, in all its guises, is an experience of the human condition and offers opportunities that either support soul development or compound loss of soul. New mother Kylie says:

> There are always consequences to our choices and actions, the cost is always paid in the kind of person we become. I wanted to transcend some old habits of my personality and develop my inner core, my soul. Because, by my choices during the birth, I was shaping myself as a mother.

So for willing women, a physical, psychological, 'spiritual growth' or capacity-building mindset offers them—even in the painful storms of labour—the motivation to *embrace* the experience rather than simply endure it.

Some women are taking normal physiological birth on as a healing journey after coming from previous birth experiences that have left them feeling wounded and traumatised.

For these women a normal physiological birth is not only about physical recovery, but also about their emotional wellbeing. Many women, like Thaïs, are left with 'a deep yearning and question in my soul and body' after the birth of a previous child. They may have felt disenfranchised in their previous birth and now, in this subsequent birth, they want to be advised of options, not dictated to; they want to be treated with respect as autonomous women. They want to stay connected, rather than being separated from their babies. They want to claim their own power for birthing and mothering.

Social awareness

Other motivations for having a go at normal physiological birth that are starting to come through from those who attend my workshops, have to do with women's values relating to social awareness. Perhaps the bike-riding, ecologically minded willing woman is going for a low-tech normal physiological birth because of the heavy ecological footprint[4] of socially 'normal' birthing. This includes the high energy use needed for technological birth, the high levels of synthetic hormones flushed into our water systems, the increased use of 'just-in-case' antibiotics, the estimated 30% of the health dollar spent on 'waste' and 'over-treatment' in health care.

Or maybe her social awareness as a global citizen may cause the willing woman to ponder the discrepancy between the average health dollar cost of her high-tech, intervention-stacked, socially normal, 'convenient and comfortable' birth experience, as compared to the experiences of her birthing sisters across the developing world.

The World Health Organization is certainly onto this issue of global health care inequity. In a 2010 study to assess the discrepancy between countries assessed as being disadvantaged by a lack of needed caesareans in comparison to countries assessed as conducting unnecessary caesareans they concluded that 'worldwide, caesarean sections that are possibly medically unnecessary appear to command a disproportionate share of global economic resources'[5], with an assessment that Australia is spending $US 37,990,115 on medically unnecessary caesareans.

Baby calling the shots

Finally, many women wishing to undertake normal physiological birth are guided by a sense of wanting to gain for herself and her baby the benefits of the human mammalian heritage of labour, birth and breastfeeding hormones.

She wants to honour her baby's birth rite—the baby's role in 'calling the shots' in its own birth. She knows that, if left to follow its own timing, the baby in utero will trigger the birth process. So the willing woman wants a normal physiological birth to allow her baby to initiate this process and to allow it to be alert and able to use its own instincts to join with her in their birth dance.

Isn't it strange that women who want all this for their baby are often accused of being selfish for wanting the 'experience' of normal physiological birth?

The right kind of motivation?

So, these are some of the motivations that women might be acting on—either consciously or unconsciously—in wishing to have a go at normal physiological labour and birth. Perhaps you recognise some of these in yourself.

They're great, but unfortunately, for many reasons, simply *wanting* a normal birth isn't enough. The most obvious reason it's not enough, of course, is that a normal physiological birth, especially with a first baby, is bloody hard work—it's not called labour for nothing!

So, in my workshops, I also ask women to try to tease out a little more about their motivations.

Given what women who want a normal physiological birth are up against in terms of the challenge of birth itself, one of the first general points I make on this issue of 'motivation' in my workshop is that a willing woman's values need to arise from within herself. She needs to be *internally* motivated.

If, instead, she's taking on a normal physiological birth because she wants to please, follow or impress someone else, or because she's still stuck in her teenage rebellion phase and wants to defy her parents or other authority figures … well, leaving aside whether these ways of being still serve her in other parts of her life, I can pretty well guarantee that this kind of motivation won't be enough to get a birthing woman through the tough gig of birthing.

During my workshops I also highlight that in many cases the motivations women give for wanting to 'have a go' at normal physiological birth are related to positive benefits expected *after* the birth.

Women talk about better bonding with their babies, about their babies not being 'drugged out', about recovering from birth more quickly. These are all good reasons, but the willing woman needs to keep in mind that, on their own, these motivations are unlikely to be enough. She's going to need some other kind of motivation to sustain her in the challenging present moments of the labour itself: in the reality of the birth experience, all those motivations to do with the future may start to feel a lot less important!

In labour, the willing woman needs to value, in some way, the physical experience of the birth process itself. She will need to find a way of engaging with that experience—perhaps by tuning into the pressure and shift in sensations that signal the movement of her baby through her body, or by noting the 'feel' quality of her body working: the stretching, opening, pushing sensations, the rhythm of her breath or instinctive rocking and spiralling movements.

It's essential she finds something she can engage with moment by moment during the tough contractions. This was certainly not a problem for Michele B, who writes:

> I want to yell and sweat. I want to feel my body heave with the power of the ages. I want to feel that almighty *fullness* again, when, in amongst the profoundly physical, I was amazed to feel the touch of divinity. And I want to experience the sweet relief of the release and the wondrous beholding of the glistening newborn that I know to be my child.

It is this ability to engage with the physical experience that will help the willing woman to stay in touch with those beliefs and values connected to future benefits—the love-bomb bonding at the birth, the health and vitality of her baby born without the compromise of a drugged-up system, the benefits of a speedier recovery (offering a better start for breastfeeding), and the strengthening of her sense of self, which will sustain her through the tough times that are bound to come over the years of parenting.

Another point I regularly emphasise is that couples need to be aware that, because normal physiological birthing is a hard gig, the values and desires that underpin a woman's decision to have a go at it need to be *lived* values. That is, they need to be values that the woman is already putting into action or that she intends to practise putting into action during pregnancy. Being inspired by some aspirational values is necessary, but basing your desire for normal physiological birth entirely on aspirational values, without any foundation in solid lived actions is … well, bound to end in tears.

If you aspire to work with functional pain in labour but never push your physical comfort zone … well? If you aspire to access your birthing instincts but wouldn't know an instinct if you fell over one … well? If you want to question your caregiver's agenda but rarely take personal responsibility for your health and wellbeing … well?

Labour-bypass era

Another reason that simply *wanting* a normal physiological birth is not enough to ensure you'll have one, is that—to my great sadness and anger—our present birth system is not set up to support normal physiological birth. More than that, it is well and truly stacked *against* this kind of birth.

In my classes, I explain to women and their partners that they are birthing in what I call the 'labour-bypass era'.

In the next chapter you'll get a better sense of what I mean by this when I take you through some of the statistics for birth in Australia. But you may already have an idea of what I'm talking about.

If you are interested in having a go at normal physiological birth—if you are a willing woman—you're probably already aware that you are out of step with the social norm when it comes to your thinking about birth. If you've voiced anything about your yearning for normal physiological birth, you've no doubt been greeted by the usual responses: 'Don't be stupid', 'You don't have to be a martyr', 'Epidurals are the way to go', 'Just you wait!'

As these reactions indicate, we are living in an era where attempting normal physiological birth is not expected, not usual, not valued, or even necessary anymore.

In this labour-bypass era birthing women no longer need to engage with their straining, striving, labouring, birthing bodies. You can have your baby without actually having to labour and birth at all, if you don't want to. Or, if you do labour, you don't have to feel it. Babies can be delivered by caesarean and bypass labour entirely, or, because of the epidural option, women can labour but bypass feeling it—you can read the Sunday paper, update your Facebook status or sleep through it.

The messages reaching women from this labour-bypass birthing culture are: healthy mother and healthy baby are all that matter, and efficient, cut and dried, convenient birthing is possible and it's your right. In fact, you definitely *should* be comfortable and pain-free.

Basically, the message is that the effort of labouring, the experience of labour and birth, has no purpose or intrinsic value.

In this labour-bypass era, the default birth is certainly not a normal physiological one, unfolding through the hormonal surges, with the birthing woman engaging with her body and her baby, supported into the work of it and reaping the hormonal rewards of the 'birth high' that bonds her to her baby.

At a time when our lifestyle aspirations encourage many of us to take advantage of more and better labour- and time-saving devices, we have now come to a place where, in ever-increasing numbers, women are being convinced they need to be saved from this kind of birth. Saved from their 'labours'.

Welcome to the labour-bypass era!

This is confronting stuff, I know, but when you look at the statistics in chapter 2 you'll see that the numbers tell the story. Fewer and fewer women are having their babies through a normal physiological birth process, and very few receive the kind of support they need to do so.

So, for now, trust me when I say that the woman who wants to undertake normal birth in Australia today needs to understand what she's up against and be prepared. She needs to understand that—whatever her motivations—platitudes about wanting a natural birth will not be nearly enough to achieve one.

When I talk to women in my workshops about the idea of a 'willing woman', I therefore differentiate between *two types* of 'willing' woman.

Firstly, there's what I call the 'naïve willing woman'. In contrast, there's what I call the 'savvy willing woman'.

I am making the assumption that in reading this book you identify yourself as a willing woman—or at the very least that you are curious about, and have some kind of yearning for, a normal physiological birth. If you do have intentions towards a normal physiological birth in this labour-bypass era, you will need to become a *savvy* willing woman.

Helping you in this transformation is the purpose of this book. The issues and choices that I will be addressing here may be of interest to any birthing woman; but they are *crucial* to those who want to have a go at normal physiological birth.

Savvy choices

One of the key differences between a naïve willing woman and a savvy one is in the nature of her choices about her birth. The choices she makes will be in response to just how much she understands about the birth process, her own attitudes, the attitudes of those around her and the birth culture of her society.

In the coming chapters I will be going into greater detail about all these influences and what they mean for your birth. For now, I am going to provide a brief overview of some important choices and ask that you begin to consider your own thoughts and feelings about these important issues. Ask yourself, how will your choices in these areas support your quest for normal physiological birth?

Place of birth

Where are you planning to have your baby—a labour ward in a large or small hospital? A city or regional hospital? A public or private hospital? A birth centre attached to a hospital? A free-standing birth centre? Or a homebirth in a mud-brick home, a triple-fronted suburban dream or an inner-city apartment? Wherever it is, what has the place of birth you are choosing got to offer you in your quest for normal physiological birth?

Does it offer proactive support for the work of labour, while also providing the appropriate level of medical attention required for the wellbeing of you and your baby? Does it offer space for movement and active birthing? Does it offer access to the natural environment? Does it offer access to a birth tub for water immersion? Does it offer warmth and privacy? In other words, does it offer the necessary elements for working with normal physiological birth?

Caregivers

Who will be the caregivers at your birth? Do they understand how to help you with the demands of normal physiological birth?

Research around the world and reported in the Cochrane database[6], suggests that women are best supported for normal physiological birth by known, experienced caregivers who are with them one on one continuously throughout labour.[7]

Ensuring you receive this kind of care is easier said than done.

In the description above, 'known' refers to having established a connection with your caregivers: having developed a trusting relationship based on a shared philosophy and vision for the birth. 'Experienced' refers to 'experience' in facilitating normal physiological birth (not just experience of birth in general). And the 'one on one continuously throughout labour' part means a caregiver continuously with you, not in and out dealing with two or three birthing women at the same time.

So the usual situation, in which hospital caregivers change shifts, strangers come in and out, a mix of rostered midwives and professionals work within hierarchical rather than collaborative structures, and where 'being with you one on one continuously in labour' is often left to the electronic fetal monitor, just doesn't cut it.

And for those who think that 'caregiver' in this latest research referred to in the Cochrane database could relate to your partner—who is known to you and shares your vision for the birth and presumably will be staying with you one on one rather than popping up and down the corridor helping other labouring women—wrong! Remember that they are not *experienced* and so don't fulfil the role recommended by this research.

The necessary combination for supporting normal physiological birth is not offered across the board in all care settings. This means willing women need to be savvy enough to hunt it down, or to design their own team by employing independent practitioners.

Because of encouragement to use private health care, over 30% of births in Australia take place in the private sector, which means many pregnant women take a path that leads them to make their primary 'known' relationship with a private obstetrician.

Being an expert in 'complex birth' doesn't mean that obstetricians are experienced in how to help you achieve an undisturbed normal physiological birth, however. In fact, the reality is very often far from it. Unfortunately, contemporary obstetric practice, through the use of techno-medical surveillance, tight timing protocols and interventions that restrict the mother, tend to disturb the physiological process. Added to that, we can see that the 'one-on-one continuously throughout labour' aspect of our ideal support is also not fulfilled by the obstetrician's role; they are not sitting with you, breathing with you, encouraging you through your contractions. This is a midwife's role.

For the willing woman to best ensure normal physiological birthing, research would strongly suggest that she make her primary connection with a midwife. In particular a 'named' midwife working with you one on one, forming a relationship with you over the pregnancy, the birth and into the early weeks of bonding and mothering—described by Professor Lesley Page, President of the Royal College of Midwives (UK) as 'a skilled companion' who accompanies you through your journey to motherhood.[8]

Very recent research from Australia (Melbourne 2012)[9] confirms the benefits of what Professor Page calls 'the development of a continuous and trusting relationship' between the mother and midwife. The research shows that pregnant women cared for in one on one caseload models (where midwives have a personal caseload of women who they make a relationship with during pregnancy, attend during birth and follow-up with post-natally), 'were more likely to avoid medical interventions during labour including caesarean sections'. This kind of care was also better for babies, reducing the need for special care after birth.[10]

Willing women need to seek out the birth situations that offer midwives as primary caregivers in caseload 'known' or 'named midwife' schemes—midwives who can make a relationship with you through your pregnancy and stay with you through the building intensity of the birth, guiding and supporting you contraction by contraction across your labour.

This is the age-old role of a midwife, which is being reclaimed by contemporary midwifery. It is described in recent midwifery theories, including 'midwifery partnership'[11], 'midwifery guardianship'[12] and 'new midwifery' models, and is framed within ideas of 'keeping birth normal'.

The 'new midwife' is skilled in knowing how to maximise your instinctive hormonal capacity; in supporting you to work with pain; in respecting your autonomy and communicating accordingly, while skilfully watching over the safety of the birthing process without disturbing it, and knowing when to access obstetric care if the birth deviates from normal parameters. This kind of care will minimise any unnecessary interventions and increase the likelihood that interventions will only be suggested for 'true medical need'.

Patient autonomy and health literacy

Understanding the range of choices is one thing, negotiating them is another. So the issue of patient autonomy and health literacy is something else that the willing woman needs to be across.

Now this is a pretty big concept, and for many of us it may be an entirely new one. What I'm talking about here is the concept of a birthing woman having the right to be informed about and say 'yes' or 'no' to medical procedures and interventions suggested to her.

It sounds fairly straightforward, right? Unfortunately though, as Associate Professor of Midwifery at University of Western Sydney Hannah Dahlen, says, '[W]omen's right to control what happens to their bodies during pregnancy and birth may be enshrined in law but this right is frequently violated in practice.'[13]

What health literacy and medical decision making *should* look like in practice is 'patient autonomy'[14] on the part of the patient—in our case the birthing woman—who will make her choices in light of the evidence provided and based on her values and research, her baby's and her own health, her sense of responsibility and her capacity.

Now her choice might either be giving 'informed consent'—that is, saying 'yes' to what's suggested; or it may be 'informed refusal'—saying 'no' to what's suggested. In either case there will be an expectation that her *autonomous choice* will be accepted without coercion or refusal of support and goodwill.

On the part of the medical caregiver, in theory they should practise in a way that honours patient autonomy and, in our case, provides the birthing woman with 'women-centred care' by sharing evidence-based information. They will quantify risk, specific to the particular woman and her baby, and practise within the code of ethics of their profession.

That is what it *should* look like. But what it more often looks like in practice is a passive patient being *informed* of what is happening. Or, in many cases, not even being informed. In fact, in order to be presented with the reason for a particular procedure or intervention the birthing woman herself may need to *ask* for this information.

The dynamic at play in these situations is what can be described as the 'trance of acquiescence'. In medical settings many of us have low levels of health literacy and may not realise that we have choice. We seem to automatically give up our autonomy and slip into this 'trance', accepting whatever is offered without discernment about whether we want it, whether we need it, or what agendas might be behind whatever is being suggested. This passive trance of acquiescence is actually the psychological equivalent of a fear-based 'freeze' state.

Because of this, interactions between medical caregivers and their patients are often transacted within this dynamic—a compliant trance of acquiescence on the part of the fearful patient, and, of course, a corresponding '*assumption* of acquiescence' on the part of the medical caregivers.

In most birthing situations this is what passes as 'informed consent'. 'The woman herself may not realise that consenting to acceptance is a choice, rather than inevitable,' explains Emeritus Professor of Midwifery at the University of Edinburgh Rosemary Mander.[15]

Added to this 'trance' and 'assumed acquiescence' dynamic, many of us are 'conflict avoidant'. We want to keep a 'good vibe' over and above speaking up for our needs in a tricky situation. Also, a tendency towards conflict avoidance is heightened in the birthing woman who is flooded with oxytocin—the loving, 'tend and befriend' hormone. She just wants to be sweet to everybody. So in the face of any tough negotiations about procedures and interventions she is more likely to fold if the environment gets tricky.

In our risk-averse, litigation-fearful birth culture, procedures and interventions useful for high-risk women and babies have increasingly become standardised as routine care for *all* mothers and babies. Willing women need to be awakened from this acculturated 'trance of acquiescence' and get savvy about the practices and procedures they will routinely be offered, in order to give 'informed consent' or—and given that these routines are designed for the worst-case scenario, more likely—to use 'informed refusal' to protect themselves from any unwanted procedures and interventions.

So, getting back to your choices, the willing woman needs not only to be aware of informed choice and consent, she also needs to be aware of her right to 'informed refusal'.

Philosophical match

These issues of patient autonomy and appropriate care bring us to the importance of ensuring you find a carer who is a good 'philosophical match' with you.

Certainly the willing woman wants to claim her autonomy and will ideally find a match with caregivers who are woman-centred in their practice. Woman-centred practitioners also want to work with women who are fully aware of the personal responsibility required of them when giving informed consent and informed refusal. This compatibility in terms of understanding patient autonomy would contribute to a philosophical match.

You can see that it would become problematic if a willing woman, aware of her need and right to exercise patient autonomy, is attended by a caregiver who is assuming acquiescence on her part. A power play generally gets going that does nothing for the birth.

Birth attendant Jess describes this situation:

> The next vaginal examination was upon us before we knew it. Karen was having very intense contractions on the bathroom floor and would not agree to move to the bed for the examination. The registrar was insisting that the vaginal examination took place on the bed.

Just as problematic would be the scenario of a woman caught up in the trance of acquiescence who wants to be told what to do, but is attended by a caregiver looking for her to take responsibility and make her own choices based on the evidence. At the very least, dissatisfaction abounds, but more problematic is a situation where these mismatches compromise safety and best-practice care.

At the core of all birth philosophies is the health and wellbeing of mothers and babies. However, as you are hopefully beginning to see by now, the emphasis on how to achieve this can vary greatly. The differences in approaches to birth stem from two very different views of birth. One view is characterised as having a general trust in birth and therefore wanting to support the physiological process. The other is characterised as distrusting birth and therefore controlling it using techno-medical processes.

As a willing woman, if you don't know whether you have a philosophical match with your (usually stranger) caregivers then you are likely to be on guard, defensive and second-guessing all the time about what the agendas are for suggesting particular procedures. You might wonder, 'Is it because there is really something wrong with me or my baby? Or is it because of some protocol required by the institution? Or is it about something else?'

Without a philosophical match, the whole scene can deteriorate into a 'this versus that' standoff, which is not great for anyone—least of all the baby. So much is dependent on ensuring that you have a philosophical match with your caregivers. This is where that 'known' caregiver bit comes in—trust comes out of an established relationship and a shared philosophy.

Conclusion

Any aspiration for normal physiological birth of course first requires that you be willing to give normal birth a go. To do this, you need to be clear about your reasons for wanting this kind of birth. Are you internally motivated or trying to impress someone else? Will any of your motivations help you through the hard physical work of labour itself, or are they all about what happens *after* the birth?

A woman's individual situation, strengths and vulnerabilities will help to determine the pathway of her birth experience. But she will also be affected by the cultural attitudes and messages—the zeitgeist—which influences behaviours and birth choices, as well as the philosophies, pressures, routines, practices and 'nudges' that hold sway in the maternity system.

Therefore, as well as being simply 'willing', the willing woman also needs to be particularly savvy because, as the next chapter will show, the Australian birthing culture is well and truly stacked against her.

In regards to the social norms of birthing, the willing woman is in the wrong place at the wrong time. So, willing woman, if you have never thought of yourself as a radical woman before, you are now.

Personal reflection

- Are you a willing woman?
- What are your motivations for working towards a normal physiological birth?
- What are the lived values that underpin your motivation?
- What aspirational values offer inspiration for normal physiological birth?
- Does the place of birth you are choosing have a culture of supporting normal birth?
- What do their statistics on inductions, caesareans, epidurals and other interventions tell you about the birth culture?
- Does the place of birth you are choosing provide access to midwifery-led care, caseload midwifery, know-your-midwife schemes or other midwifery initiatives to maximise possibilities for keeping birth normal?
- What is your level of health literacy?
- What is your capacity for negotiating 'informed consent' or 'informed refusal' decisions?
- Do you have a philosophical match with your caregivers?

2

Reality hurts: birth in the labour-bypass era

If you're pregnant and you've told your friends and family about it, or you're starting to show, you're probably starting to hear some birth stories by now—from your girlfriends or your aunts, your mother, the woman down the shops, at work or at the hairdresser. It's amazing how all the stories come out, a testament to our human desire for sharing and wanting to connect.

Now, unless you're very lucky—and I'd have to say unusual—you will have begun to hear, among all these birth experiences, some 'thank goodness' stories. You know, those stories where things went wrong and 'Thank goodness the obstetrician was there,' 'Thank goodness we could get the caesarean,' 'Thanks goodness for the forceps,' 'for the vacuum extraction,' 'for the induction'.

These stories are everywhere and they make birth seem like quite a tricky business. They might also make you think that you are pretty likely to end up needing that caesarean or those forceps or that vacuum extraction yourself.

Well, unless you're savvy, the chances are that you will have some kind of intervention during your birth, but not necessarily because you or your baby *need* it.

When I hear these 'thank goodness' stories, I am deeply saddened because I know that the vast majority of these interventions—this 'saving' by the hospital, the obstetrician, the midwife—are not necessary. Or at least that they weren't necessary to start with and very likely only became necessary as a result of earlier unnecessary routine procedures and interventions.

I'm saddened because I know that, more often than not, the mother and baby have experienced unnecessary interference in their birth, resulting in these unintended consequences. And because I know that the birthing woman who experienced these interventions has no idea that things could have gone a different way.

Things *can* go a different way when a pregnant woman, as well as wanting to have a normal birth, has the information to help her realistically prepare for it. Today, the *savvy willing woman* needs to know what she's up against—that is, that she's attempting labour in a labour-bypass era.

Birthing against the odds

If you're aware of the stats for birth, you may already have worked out that in Australia at the present time, especially if you're having your first baby, you're as likely to have a surgical intervention as not. If not a caesarean, then at least a vacuum extraction or forceps will be used to birth your baby.

For some of you, because of medical complexity, that will be exactly what you and your baby need, and for some women it's what they choose. But I also know that there are some of you who are regretful or sadly resigned to this probability, and that there are still others for whom the knowledge that it could come down to (or has already come down to) this, is deeply distressing.

You're birthing at a time when caesareans have come to rule the roost. Their prevalence means that all other types of birth—non-caesarean births—are defined in contrast to them. So we now talk about either caesarean or 'normal' birth.

But don't be fooled by this use of the term 'normal'. We're not talking about physiologically normal. Indeed, most of these 'non-caesarean' births are anything but. They include vacuum extractions and forceps and inductions and epidurals and episiotomies and more. The only sense in which most of them could be understood as 'normal' is if we're talking about *socially* normal. Because in the current birth scene, interventions are so prevalent they've certainly become the social norm.

In Australia at present, it's very easy for you to access an intervention-stacked birth. I don't mean easy in the sense that you will cruise through it; I use the word easy in the sense that interventions—whether routinely administered, socially chosen or medically necessary—are readily available. They, including all those caesareans, are now the default option. As Associate Professor of Midwifery at University of Western Sydney Hannah Dahlen says: 'A first-time mother in Australia now has a greater chance of having surgical intervention during her birth than not having it.'[16]

Is this normal?

Perhaps you're thinking this is a pretty normal and reasonable state of affairs. Well, let's have a look at Australia's stats in a broader perspective. The World Health Organization (WHO) did a study some years ago to assess appropriate levels of interventions for 'true medical need'.[17] Their results suggested, for example, that no country in the world would need an induction rate over 10%, or a caesarean rate greater than 10–15%.

Overall in Australia, according to the most recently released figures (Australia's Mothers and Babies Report, 2014)[18], we have an induction rate of around 28%, and a caesarean rate over 33% (with some hospitals above 50%). So you can see there seems to be something other than 'true medical need' at play here.

In Australia, in addition to the high caesarean and induction rates, we have a vacuum extraction rate of 11%; forceps rate of 8%; augmentation rate (speeding up the labour) of 16% of all births and overall pain-relief rate of 77% (with an 87% rate in first births). Troubling as these statistics might seem, the figures are even more confronting on closer look. Looking at augmentation (speeding up the birth), for example: when we remove the 48% of births that do not start spontaneously because they are induced (28%) or elective caesareans (20%), we are left with a 'spontaneous onset of labour' rate of 51%. Of these spontaneous onset births, 31% will go on to be augmented.

Added to all these figures, managed third stage (the use of synthetic hormones to deliver the placenta) is, apart from in small pockets, practically standard across the board.

You do the maths. Not too many mums and babies are getting through without some form of intervention.

It's worth noting that rates for all interventions have been increasing, so presumably, given the two-year time lag in producing birth statistics, the intervention rates are now even higher than I'm reporting here. Also, these figures are for all births; they are generally higher across the board for first births.

Even so, you may be lulled into thinking it's not too bad here if you mistakenly believe that the figures for 'spontaneous vaginal birth' (54%) equate to a figure for 'normal physiological birthing'. Unfortunately this is not the case.

That 'spontaneous vaginal birth' statistic only refers to births where the baby emerges through the vagina instead of being assisted by using forceps or vacuum extraction, or through a caesarean delivery. In other words, these figures don't mean that no other interventions have been used. They certainly don't mean that the physiologically normal hormonal dance between mother and baby has unfolded.

Instead, these spontaneous vaginal birth figures can include synthetic hormones for inductions and augmentations, artificial rupture of membranes, continuous electronic fetal monitoring, scalp electrodes, catheters, 'just in case' antibiotics, all the drugs and procedures for pain relief, episiotomy, and synthetic hormone-managed third stage.

Interestingly, even this term 'spontaneous vaginal birth'—which at least alludes to something approaching normal physiological process—has, since 2007, been changed to 'non-instrumental vaginal birth', reflecting the labour-bypass culture's 'intervention as the norm' bias.

Not a level playing field

Now, it's important to point out that, although I'm giving you the overall Australian birth figures, intervention rates vary in different settings, from state to state, public to private hospitals and birth-setting to birth-setting.

Many pregnant women assume that it is a level playing field out there. They assume that if they ended up with an induction, an epidural, a caesarean or any of the other interventions, it was because it was medically necessary. They assume that regardless of where they had their baby, the same outcome would have eventuated. Unfortunately this is far from the case. It's not a level playing field out there.

For example, in the event that the waters break as the first sign of a woman's impending labour without her yet experiencing any contractions, the likelihood of a resulting intervention will depend on where her birth is taking place and under whose care. In some settings, if you haven't gone into labour within 12–24 hours, an induction is advised, while in other settings (in the absence of any other concerning factors) the protocols of the hospital or specific caregivers could mean waiting 48 hours and, in some cases, as long as 72 hours before considering an induction. Obviously, the more expansive the time frame in a place of birth, the less likely an induction will be needed, meaning more women at that place of birth will spontaneously go into labour.

The public versus private hospital choice can be a confusing one for willing women who are not aware of the statistics. Many make the seemingly logical assumption that the quality of care they receive in a private hospital will be superior to that in a public hospital. However, all private hospitals have higher rates of medical interventions during birth than public hospitals; for instance, the rate for 'non-instrumental vaginal births' is 59% in pubic hospitals, and 42% in private hospitals, while the rate for caesarean births is 29% in public hospitals and 43% in private hospitals (Australia's Mothers and Babies Report, 2014).[19] This can be counter-intuitive, because generally very high-risk women and babies go to our tertiary-level public hospitals, which are equipped with neo-natal intensive care units. You might therefore think that the intervention rates at these public hospitals would be higher, but no, they're not.

This is supported by an Australian study recently published in the British Medical Journal's online journal, *BMJ Open*, as reported in the *Age* newspaper: 'In a landmark study of nearly 700,000 women in New South Wales' hospitals, those giving birth privately were found to have a 20% lower chance of delivering their first child through normal vaginal birth.'[20] Professor Hannah Dahlen of the University of Western Sydney, who led the study, added: 'We looked at the healthiest, wealthiest population possible, exploding some of the myths out there that women receiving these interventions are sicker.'[21]

If normal physiological birth is important to you—your choice of birth place matters.

What about other countries?

There are countries that fit more closely with the WHO recommendations on interventions than Australia. These are generally countries, such as the UK, that have continued a legacy of midwives as primary caregivers for healthy, low-risk pregnant women with uncomplicated births—with obstetricians providing specialist back-up only for complex, high-risk pregnancy and births. Erin's story from the Maternity Coalition's *Birth Matters Journal* illustrates this difference. Erin said:

> We arrived in England and soon realised that we had stumbled across a very different birthing culture to that of Melbourne. As I began to receive emails from home asking me if I had chosen an obstetrician or hospital yet, we had our first meeting at our local GP's surgery. This GP warmly told us that I wasn't ill, that in the

> UK pregnancy was considered a normal life stage and that my care would be provided by a midwife. The following week we met our midwife, Jan, who came to our tiny flat for the first of many home visits. At our home visit at thirty weeks Jan ran through our birthing choices: I could either have a homebirth or birth in the midwife-led unit at the hospital.[22]

Such maternity care systems are backed by Iain Chalmers, Murray Enkin and Marc Kierse who concluded in *Effective Care in Pregnancy and Childbirth*, a systematic review of the worldwide literature on childbirth practices, that 'it is inherently unwise and perhaps unsafe, for women with normal pregnancies to be cared for by obstetric specialists, even if the required personnel are available'.[23]

The approach in countries like the UK is distinct from Australia, where the default option is to use obstetricians as primary caregivers, especially if you have private health cover.

Upon returning to Australia in 2005 Erin was surprised by her experience of her second pregnancy.

> I was completely flummoxed by the disjointed system in Australia. The first GP I saw assumed I had my own obstetrician and was totally confused by my asking how I could access continuous care by midwives.

According to obstetrician Euan Wallace, Director of Obstetric Services, Southern Health, one of the challenges in Australia is that: 'looking after healthy pregnancies is the bread and butter for a large section of the obstetric workforce'.[24] In other words, despite the evidence that obstetric care does not result in the best outcomes for low-risk women, there are many with vested interests in maintaining it as the norm in Australia.

There are countries with outcomes for mothers and babies that are comparable to or better than Australia, but with lower intervention rates. Sweden has maternal and perinatal outcomes that are equal to Australia's but with half the number of interventions. Our neighbours in New Zealand enjoy a restructured maternity system where midwives are more likely to be the primary caregivers, and where they have kept their caesarean rate at 20%, compared to our 33%.[25]

There are countries with the same kinds of social, cultural and lifestyle pressures that influence the way women give birth here in Australia, but in many of these countries frameworks have been put in place specifically to support normal physiological birth at a structural level. Examples include the Keeping Childbirth Natural and Dynamic (KCND) Program (Scotland 2009); All Wales Clinical Pathway for Normal Labour (Wales 2002–04); and also in the UK: 'Changing Childbirth' the Royal College of Midwives Campaign for Normal Birth and 'National Institute for Clinical Excellence' (NICE Guidelines).[26] [27]

Normal physiological birthing: an endangered activity

'Normal physiological birthing'. I use this phrase a lot and it sounds clumsy I know, but I repeat it as often as I can—because it's become an endangered human activity.

Perhaps it's telling in itself, but there is no category for normal physiological birth in the statistics. Instead, we have to try to infer it.

One way of teasing out these statistics is to add together the figures for births we can assume approach normal physiological birth because of their setting—those in birth centres (set up for low-risk women to support normal physiological birth) (1.8%); home births (0.3%); and the 'born before arrivals' —you know, those babies born on the back seats of cars and on doorsteps (0.4%). Added together, these figures suggest normal physiological births make up only about 3% of all current births.

Another way I try to get an idea of the normal physiological birth figures is by asking midwives about it when I present seminars in hospitals. I ask 'What percentage of normal physiological birth happens in this hospital?' After initial haggling about whether they can include this or that intervention in the normal physiological figures (which I politely refuse, emphasising that I want 'just normal physiological birth') the range midwives give is somewhere between 1 and 5%.

What's going on?

Why are our intervention rates so high?

Even though the physiological birthing process itself hasn't changed across eons of human development, it is subject to cultural influences. And certainly, as a result of broader shifts in cultural expectations and lifestyle, what we currently think and do about birth in this labour-bypass era has changed.

The spirit of the age, the cultural currents at play, the zeitgeist: call it what you like, it shapes our thoughts, expectations and behaviours, both generally and around birth.

One cultural current at play is the way our motivations for accessing medical interventions more broadly have shifted from 'medical need' to 'social choice' and onto 'social expectation'.

A couple's story some years ago alerted me to the extent of these shifts in social expectations in the realm of birth. This couple had come to me in very late pregnancy to sort through an issue to do with the father's parents. These parents, the grandparents-to-be, had come from interstate for the birth and now, as the baby was overdue, they wanted the mother-to-be to have her labour induced before they had to return to Perth. They were putting pressure on her, via their son. They couldn't understand why their daughter-in-law wouldn't agree because, as they said, 'We know lots of women who have had inductions, it's no big deal'. Well, maybe it wasn't a big deal for them but for this pregnant woman it was certainly a very big deal.

Her partner's parents felt that her refusal to be induced was a slight to them as grandparents. Their thinking was shaped by the cultural currents. They were coming from a socially normalised position regarding induction and felt it wasn't very important how the baby was born. The pregnant woman, on the other hand, was a willing woman, coming from an understanding of the importance of normal physiological birthing and to her it most certainly *did* matter how the baby was born.

Now, a few years later, given the increased trend towards elective caesareans, I wonder if the pressure would be on for the woman to have a caesarean to accommodate her in-laws or anyone else for that matter.

Convenience above all

Our busy, pressured lifestyles don't serve pregnant or birthing women very well. The necessarily 'slowed down' tuning in, the 'graciously waiting upon' character of both late pregnancy, normal physiological birth and the early post-natal period, are at odds with lifestyles that push us, faster and faster, to expect results and outcomes.

So much of our technology drives an expectation of immediacy—measured in milliseconds, with an equally immediate rise in frustration if that expectation is not met. After all, does your computer ask you to chill out and slow down? So, our instant-gratification lifestyle is diminishing our tolerance for waiting on processes to unfold ... how might that play out in birthing? Well, I think the rise in inductions, augmentations and caesareans is all part of it.

Wanting convenience in all things increasingly influences cultural expectations across the board. We want it now, we want it here, we don't want to be put out. We want it on tap. So what might the convenient 'on demand' birth look like? One where you can plan when it will happen, how long it might take, how comfortable you should be ... I'm sure you can begin to imagine.

Mini baby boom

You are also birthing at a time when the so-called mini baby boom of the past few years shows no sign of abating (there were 55,000 more babies born in 2014 than there were in 2004, an 18% rise), putting our hospitals and birthing systems under stress. The pressure of getting you in, getting you out, and freeing up beds, is also adding to the 'fast' birth expectations on the part of our hospitals.

Perhaps it's not surprising then that there can often be a blurring of agendas. 'Convenience' and 'fast-birth' agendas on the part of the caregiver or place of birth can often be presented to birthing women in terms of medical risk. New mother Jinni explains:

> After being told that it was 'risky' to go past due date, when we asked the obstetrician to quantify the risk, he could not do so. Then he asked, had we considered an elective caesarean? Given that an induction probably wouldn't work, he thought that this might be the wisest—and least problematic—course of action. Least problematic for whom, we thought?

Maybe the almost-standard use of synthetic hormones to manage third stage is another case in point. Although recommended to control blood loss (and required for true medical need in some cases) it also has a time-saver 'benefit'. The timeline for routinely managed third stage is ten to twenty minutes and involves an injection of synthetic oxytocin to the mother as the baby's head is being born, followed by cord traction, fundal pressure and rush, rush to get the placenta 'task' ticked off. In contrast, in care settings still practising normal physiological birthing, third stage (where the birthing of the placenta is triggered by the natural hormones released at birth and boosted by the baby nuzzling and initiating breastfeeding) can take up to forty-five minutes. During this time the undisturbed mother and baby are taking the early steps of their hormonally directed dance of bonding. So, who benefits from the time-saver of synthetic hormone-managed third stage? I don't think it's generally the mother and baby.

Culture of risk

In many areas of life we are seeing the effects of the combined trend towards increased risk-aversion and a litigation-fearful culture, leading to the 'worst case dictates all behaviour' or what's called 'dread' risk scenarios. In birthing, this results in situations that are often laughable—for instance, a birthing woman going into hospital and not being allowed to take in a hot water bottle (so helpful for comfort and aching backs) in case she burns herself with it and then sues the hospital.

Other situations that result from this risk-aversion and litigation-fearful mindset can undermine a woman's physiological birthing capacity; for instance, the routine use of continuous electronic monitoring of the baby's heartbeat. Called an 'admission trace' or 'baseline reading', this has become routine practice in our birthing rooms, even though there is no evidence that it is helpful in healthy low-risk pregnancy.

It's assumed that birthing women will comply with the suggestion when they first arrive in hospital, to 'just pop up on the bed'. 'We'll just strap these electrodes on you, just be still so we can get a good twenty-minute trace on this baby,' they're told. But not only is there no evidence this is helpful for low-risk women and babies, research actually shows that, for these women and babies, in comparison to using intermittent heartbeat checks (doppler or sonicaid), this use of routine continuous electronic fetal monitoring results in more caesarean and instrumental deliveries, with *no added benefit* shown for the wellbeing of babies.[28]

As sociologist Raymond DeVries in his book *A Pleasing Birth*[29] says:

> Study after study showed the same thing. Electronic fetal monitoring (EFM) had one, and only one, striking effect: It raised the rate of caesarean sections. It had no effect on the health of mothers and babies. The evidence was so overwhelming that the American College of Obstetricians and Gynecologists formally recommended that routine EFM be discontinued. This advice had little effect: Today EFM accompanies over 80 percent of births in America.

And we would have to say its use is also sky-high in Australia, where, at least in my home city of Melbourne, an admissions trace is standard in most hospitals. 'Fucking madness,' says new mother Leigh. 'You can't even get through emergency to get up to the birthing unit without having one of these!'

This routine use of an 'admissions trace' for low-risk mothers and babies is not warranted for medical safety but rather for the hospital's medico-legal considerations. For the savvy willing woman it is definitely an 'informed refusal' opt-out situation.

In our risk-averse, litigation-fearful birth culture, dominated as it is by the worst-case scenario, interventions that are genuinely useful for high-risk women and babies have increasingly become standardised as routine care for *all* mothers and babies. Some women are aware that the routine practices arising from this risk paradigm are not supportive of their birthing potential, and that if they want to attempt normal physiological birth they will need to polish up their 'informed refusal' skills.

Of course, in doing this birthing women need to take into account guidance from trusted caregivers with a philosophical match with their own intentions about their birth. And they need to be aware of any individual risk factors that may apply to their particular situation. But the birthing woman *does* have the right to reject routine practices influenced by the 'medico-legal monster', as one mother named it.

Unfortunately, many women are not aware of either the likely effects of the risk-averse birth culture, or of their ability to 'opt out' of it. The 'trance of acquiescence' dynamic mentioned in chapter 1 takes over and women go along with the default option of interventions originally designed for a minority of high-risk birthing women.

In their book *Your Medical Choices: how to decide what is right for you*, medical practitioners Jerome Groopman and Pamela Hartzband confirm this default effect: 'Research in behavioural psychology shows that most people will accept the default option; they assume that what is routinely recommended is "best". It takes effort for a non-expert to decline the default option and seek an alternative.'[30]

Pathways to interventions

Australia's high-intervention birth culture, while being influenced by the many factors above, has been enabled by advancements in anaesthetics—especially epidurals—as well as medical technology and surgery techniques making caesareans faster and less problematic.

In the main, these are excellent developments and we wouldn't want to be without them. But, as the disparity between our figures and the WHO's guidelines for interventions show, they are used far more often than appears necessary for true medical need. So what's going on? What pathways might lead to these interventions?

True medical need

Obviously a percentage of birth interventions are required for true medical need and we are privileged in Australia to have ready access to these interventions. Sometimes these interventions are necessary because of the mother's or baby's high-risk health status before labour, or because of difficulties occurring during the birth itself. In these situations, even those savvy willing women wholeheartedly committed to a normal physiological birth would, if convinced of the medical necessity, accept these needed interventions.

Circumstantial interventions

These are the interventions—often unintended by the woman—that arise because they are routine for the institution or the caregiver. They are a consequence of routine protocols or 'bundles' of interventions devised by the hospitals to standardise clinical procedures. I call these 'package deal' births or (and I may be showing my age here) 'Sussan' births. Some of you may remember the clothing chain's old jingle 'this goes with that'? Well, I'm talking about 'this goes with that' births—induction goes with epidural, goes with vacuum extraction, goes with episiotomy, goes with managed third stage. Or induction goes with epidural, goes with emergency caesarean, goes with breastfeeding difficulties. These are 'cascade of intervention' births.

These circumstantial interventions have been standardised for the place of birth rather than individualised for the mother's or baby's circumstances. The episiotomy I received during the birth of my first baby illustrates this circumstantial pathway. Remember I discovered that, of the twelve women on my postnatal ward after my first daughter's birth, ten had had episiotomies and two had had caesareans! I had the same feeling as this woman after her more recent birth ended in a caesarean:

> I had a sense that it was just one long operation in there and every now and then, they would just change women, like a sausage factory.

What shapes these routines and standardised protocols ending in 'Sussan' births? Well, certainly medical safety considerations are part of it, but these routines are also influenced by the fact that hospitals are businesses, institutions, workplaces. Occupational health and safety, staffing and shift-work issues, litigious culture and defensive-practice influences (not to mention insurance companies and 'big pharma' pressures on obstetric styles) all serve to shape the protocols that end in a 'cascade of interventions'.

It also bears mentioning again here that these routine practices and protocols are not necessarily the same across all settings and caregivers. It is not a level playing field and, surprising as it is to some, these protocols are not always governed by best-practice research, so there's great variety. Again, if normal physiological birth is important to you—your choices matter.

Nudge birthing

Then we have 'nudge birthing', which relates to the issue of choice. Really, I feel we should think of birth choices as being either 'savvy', aware choices—or 'nudge' choices. Some of you may be familiar with Richard Thaler and Cass Sunstein's 'nudge' concept.[31] If not, you'll certainly be familiar with the nudge effect because marketing relies on it, nudging us this way and that, with surgical precision, through conscious and unconscious manipulation.

The nudge effect can work in an ad hoc manner, or it can be skilfully designed to influence behaviour by focusing our attention in particular directions.

According to 'nudge' understandings, in any situation where we have to make a choice there is no such thing as a neutral base. In the birth world, obstetricians, midwives and any others advising you about birth—me included—are all what Thaler and Sunstein call 'choice architects'. The way we provide you with information is either intentionally or inadvertently designed to shape your choice. So the credibility you ascribe to us, and the status and power we hold, will influence your choice-making.

Remember, too, that default options act as powerful nudges. In terms of a nudge, an 'opt-out' choice design (needing to take steps to opt-out of the default setting or situation) is particularly effective as it relies partly on the power of inertia. Whenever it's more hassle to say no and easier to comply there's a nudge at work. Junk mail, unsolicited marketing phone calls and spam, as well as many banking, phone and technology contracts, for instance, operate this way. You're stuck with them unless you actively take steps to opt-out—and the opt-out procedures are complex and time consuming.

Present birth culture is like this. You are funnelled along, nudged along the routine procedures and intervention pathways whether you want it or not—unless you are discerning enough to opt-out of the nudge. And even then you've usually got a fight on your hands.

Social choice

Birthing, as I've remarked earlier, is not isolated from more general societal shifts. In recent years we have seen that many medical procedures that were first developed for 'true medical need' have been taken up as 'social choice' and then sometimes even slid into the realm of 'social expectation'. For instance, plastic surgery techniques developed for deformities, burn and accident victims—that is, for true medical need—have now morphed into being a social-choice option for those who have the money or desire. And in some situations they have slipped even further—into the realm of social expectation. You know: the expectation that if you are a woman (or man for that matter) of a 'certain age' you *should* have your eyes done or face lifted or you'll be considered a loser in the ageing stakes.

In this high-intervention birth culture a similar drift has occurred in birthing. Inductions, for instance, were developed to aid babies who were compromised by overstaying their time in their mother's womb. But they have shifted into a social-choice option for convenience and planning on the part of the mother or her partner, or to suit the obstetric or hospital schedules. (So much so that clusters of births that used to occur in rhythm with the natural world—new and full moon, high tides, storms—now often cluster on Tuesdays and late Friday afternoons, making them convenient for the working week and for hospital workloads.)

Induction and now even elective caesareans are morphing further into social expectation—the expectation that perhaps a labour *should* be induced, or a caesarean done to aid convenience all round. After all, in our jam-packed lives, surely all this patiently waiting on the baby's timing to trigger the labour at some unpredictable point across a four-week range (two weeks either side of the due date) is just too inconvenient and frustrating? Surely it's better all round to plan it!

It's no surprise then that some inductions, or elective caesareans, while not being medically necessary, are nonetheless actively chosen by the mother for social reasons. For instance, to make the baby's birth date more convenient for her work, or her partner, or extended family responsibilities. Some women who make these choices do so with full knowledge of the likely 'cascade of intervention' consequences, while other women who make these choices may not have full awareness of the implications of their decision—of the fact that a cascade of further intervention or unexpected outcomes will usually go with the induction or elective caesarean 'package'.

Unfortunately, not many women are aware that, as the Health at a Glance OECD 2011 report reminds us, 'caesarean delivery continues to result in increased maternal mortality, maternal and infant morbidity and increased complications for subsequent deliveries'.[32] In other words, even though they are safer than they used to be, caesareans shouldn't be undertaken without serious consideration, and it's probably best if they're not offered lightly, as part of a 'birth choice smorgasbord'.

There's also the 'chicken or egg' argument between 'nudge birthing' suggestions on the part of caregivers, and 'social-choice' options on the part of the pregnant woman—which comes first? Do caregivers construct their protocols because of what women want, or are women's social choices influenced by caregivers' nudges or social and cultural expectations?

It's sometimes surprising how social pressures and expectations can take their toll on the resolve of even those women who are aware of them and want to resist.

Pain pathways

Finally, there's the pain pathway to interventions. A comfortable, pain-free, pain-relief mindset, backed by drugs and medical procedures, is currently at the centre of Australia's birth culture. Buying into this mindset, either consciously or as a subliminal acculturation, leads the majority of birthing women to go for the drugs. Or, more specifically these days, the epidural.

These drugs are interventions in their own right, but they also become the common entry point for a further cascade of interventions when the side-effects of these pain-relief options need to be counter-acted. For instance, epidurals increase the rates of vacuum extraction, because the birthing woman can no longer feel and therefore can no longer respond effectively to her 'bearing down' urge; or they can lead to caesarean deliveries because some babies don't seem to appreciate the epidural and their heartbeats then show signs of distress. The Cochrane Collaboration reported that epidurals often begin the cascade that leads to the increased need for surgical intervention to complete the birth.[33]

This pain pathway is an incredibly important one for a birth's outcome and I'm going to discuss it further in the coming chapters. For now, you can see how attitudes to pain influence our intervention rates.

These are some of the pathways to intervention. We can all agree that the first—true medical need—is a necessary pathway. But what about the others? Well, many of the previously mentioned 'thank goodness' births happen as unintended outcomes of these other pathways. Couples often don't realise that most of the 'baby saving' that was required was *because* of what was set in play by earlier routine procedures, nudge choices and pain-relief options. Unintended interventions they may have been, but hardly unpredictable when you understand the present labour-bypass era birth culture.

Because of all these different pathways to interventions (true medical need, circumstantial, nudge, social choice and pain), it becomes very difficult for the willing woman to discern, in the pressure-cooker atmosphere of a birth, whether any suggested interventions are really medically necessary for her or her baby here and now, or arise because of other pathways.

Where's the love bomb? Birthing without hormones

What saddens me about Australia's unnecessarily high intervention rates is what women and their babies are missing out on. Most women giving birth in Australia today miss out on a naturally unfolding hormone-driven birth—and all the (often downplayed) benefits this kind of birth will bring.[34]

An unintended consequence of our current birth culture is that many births do not end up relying on either the baby's or the mother's hormonal input. Ideally in birth, the baby and mother share a connected dance of readiness and response. Hormonally, the baby triggers the birth, initiating its own birth timing: the mother responds, and their birth dance begins.

In Australia, if we add together the births that use synthetic hormones to artificially kick-start them (induction, 28%) or get the hurry-up (augmentation, 16%) and the babies delivered by 'elective' caesarean with no labour at all (20%), then we have 64% of babies definitely not calling the shots on the timing of their births.

Added to this is the huge number of vaginal births in which the final oxytocin surge or 'love bombing' in third stage is overridden by an injection of synthetic oxytocin. These intervention rates mean we have a majority of births occurring with neither baby nor mother fully following their own instinctive rhythms or being exposed to the full blast of our evolutionarily programmed love and bonding hormones.

Does this mean anything? Does this mean anything for the baby, that from the start of its life it is not in rhythm with itself? Does it mean anything that the mother and baby are not sharing the hormonal cocktail of normal physiological birth? Does it mean anything that at a societal level so many births occur without any love hormones, let alone the full 'love bomb' hormonal cocktail?

Does it matter that in such high numbers of births natural oxytocin is replaced by drips of synthetic oxytocin (which, while able to drive contractions, doesn't cross the blood-brain barrier and therefore doesn't initiate bonding behaviours)? That in so many births pethidine and epidural anaesthesia replace natural endorphins and intense human support? That synthetic oxytocin delivers the placenta, replacing the surge of natural oxytocin that facilitates bonding and loving connections?

Well, social anthropologists, physiology researchers and neurobiologists say it means a lot. And so do many of the mothers who have unwittingly ended up with one of these 'no love hormone' births. Much of the new discipline of neurobiology takes as its basic premise the importance of our species' need for social connectedness (read oxytocin) and empathy. In other words—love. They don't specifically look at what happens during birth, but they do look at the earliest interactions of babies with their carers, generally mothers. They take as their starting point this early infant period and the absolute need for the human infant to be securely attached to nurturing caregivers for its ongoing physical, mental and relational 'thriving'. They know that the quality of our early interactions and nurturing (or not) affect our biology.

So if, in our era of high interventions, we so regularly interfere with the physiological, biological basis of the capacity for early bonded interactions in both the mother and the baby … what might be the implications?

A number of birth writers and researchers, including Michel Odent, are pondering these implications. Odent poses this as an 'unprecedented turning point in the history of mankind'.[35]

Conclusion

By now you will hopefully have a sense of the kind of birth our current culture shapes—the default birth in this labour-bypass era. It's one that is overwhelmingly likely to include interventions of some kind, even when the interventions are not for true medical need. It is one that increasingly seems likely to end in a caesarean section—and again, not always or even often due to medical need.

That's the reality you're facing, and maybe there are birthing women happy with the high intervention rates that are a consequence of this labour-bypass era. But if you are a willing woman interested in anything approaching normal physiological birth you have an uphill battle on your hands.

Understanding this will hopefully help you to make wise choices about your place of birth and caregivers. Hopefully, too, understanding that you're up against the labour-bypass era will motivate you to flex your informed 'opt-out' muscle.

But even with a good working knowledge of Australia's birth culture, there is one thing above all else that you will need to get right in order to have a go at normal physiological birth—and that is your attitude to pain.

Personal reflection

- Have you been hearing many 'thank goodness' birth stories?
- Now that you have some understanding of our birth culture, can you view these stories in a different light?
- Have you researched the intervention rates in your chosen place of birth?
- Have you researched your caregiver's intervention rates?
- How savvy are you about the 'nudge effect' on other choices in your life?
- Can you apply this understanding to your birthing choices?

3

It's a fine line: reframing pain in labour

In this chapter I'm going to explore the role of pain in childbirth—the cultural attitudes to this pain, the way we're programmed to deal with it during the labour, and, ultimately, the importance of reframing your view of pain in the context of birth.

Before we get into any serious discussion about pain in labour though, let me say a word on swearing.

As an educator, I usually half-heartedly apologise for swearing so readily in my workshops when I talk about birthing, and so I apologise now in advance to my readers. My excuse for swearing is that I've been hanging out with birthing women for far too long and they swear. Sometimes a lot. Why, you ask? Research has been done that has found swearing in particular (not just using any words or sounds with gusto, but actual swearing) gives some pain relief.

It worked for birthing woman Krissy during the major contractions of late first stage with her second baby. As the contraction built to a peak, with building gusto across the contraction, she responded with this song: 'It's intense, it's very intense, it's very, very intense, it's *fucking intenssssse*, it's coming down, it's finishing now, it's finishing now, it's finishing.' A very effective 'working with pain' technique!

So, I do apologise for swearing, but as I said, it's half-hearted—because if you're preparing for labour you just might need to get used to it!

Birth as peak performance

There is power in women's bodies and they give expression to this power in a glorious abundance of activities and endeavours. The dancer, athlete, aerial performer, swimmer, runner, mountain climber, yoga practitioner—all push beyond their existing comfort zones, experiencing their bodies in the intensity of personal-best, peak-performance activities.

To express this power they are challenged to work with pain, to get friendly with pain—the functional pain of their bodies straining and striving.

We are often inspired and awed by this power and potency when we celebrate it as peak bodily performance and achievement—or episodes of 'superior functioning', as these experiences have been described by one sports psychologist.[36] Effort-filled and often painful, these episodes are expressions of our body working towards behaviours that exceed our average performance. We celebrate all that we know has gone into the achievement: the determination, the commitment, the skill, the work, the hours—the *pain*.

We *know* it takes *working with pain* to achieve peak performance of the human body. In celebrating the triumph of the swimmer, the dancer, the athlete, we are also acknowledging what it has taken that swimmer, dancer and athlete, to get there—pain and all!

Acceptance of 'functional pain' goes with this territory of physical achievement and power. By 'functional pain' I am referring to the physiological pain felt in a healthy body working at high intensity, well beyond usual comfort levels. I am *not* talking about the pathological pain that arises from injury or disease.

While we accept this pain in any number of other situations, and are generally in awe of people who push through it for achievement, unfortunately acceptance of functional, physiological pain often gets lost when it comes to birthing.

We have lost an appreciation for the painful sensations birthing women experience when their bodies are labouring to release their babies—muscles working, twitching and straining; stretch receptors burning to the max; the 'drawing up' and dragging pull of muscle fibres opening the cervix.

Birthing women's ligaments are stretching to allow the hips to splay and pelvis to open to release the baby. They are experiencing burn and backache as the coccyx is pressed outward to make space for the baby to descend; their diaphragm, abs and core muscles engage to add power to the contracting uterus in second stage as they bear down to bring their baby into their arms; they sweat and strain with the effort to keep their breathing going, to keep it regular. All that full-on physiological effort and functional pain are the result of the peak performance of a woman's labouring, birthing body.

But far from celebrating this engagement with the physiological pain as an expression of a birthing woman's power and achievement, we pity her. We feel that she's suffering needlessly and want to save her from the experience.

In our culture, we have placed childbirth almost entirely in a medical context and this influences our attitudes to labour pain. Pain in a medical context is generally viewed as suffering and associated with illness, injury, things going wrong or conditions getting worse. Pain in childbirth has therefore, by default, also become associated with this negative 'suffering' context, rather than being seen in connection to satisfaction in bodily power, peak performance and achievement.

Reframing pain

While I acknowledge that some of us regularly engage with the functional pain of our bodies working, in the main we come from a pain-avoiding, comfort-obsessed culture, fearful of pain and out of practice in how to deal with it, apart from by using a plethora of pain-relieving drugs.

According to Richard Smith, from addiction service the Raymond Hader Clinic, as reported in the *Sunday Age*, Australians are 'the highest per capita users of analgesics (paracetamol and aspirin) in the world'.[37] We all appear to have a 'painkiller' mindset. So the willing woman has her work cut out for her because our cultural attitudes to pain mean that the 'nudge' is certainly towards the drugs.

Over the past decade or so there has been a pendulum swing away from any acceptance of working with pain in labour. This shift has been accelerated by ready access to epidurals and has swept us towards expectations of 'pain-free' birthing.

Today, as well as the birthing women who specifically seek out epidurals for a pain-free experience, many other women who are influenced by this painkiller/pain-free mindset go on the elusive 'mind over matter' quest for a pain-free birth. You know—the 'if we don't call it pain it won't be painful' idea. This thinking surfaced in the late seventies when I trained as a childbirth educator and has come back around. I thought it was off the mark then and I haven't been persuaded differently since.

Back when I began teaching childbirth education there was psychoprophylaxis, a rigorous, complicated breathing regime that promised 'painless childbirth'. Currently, 'Hypnobirthing'[38], 'Calm Birth' and even 'Orgasmic Birth'[39] hopefuls may be lulled into expectations of pain-free ecstatic experiences. Now I'm not saying that this isn't possible, but for a first birth it's not probable. If it's a second or subsequent birth after a normal physiological experience for your first, then your odds of fulfilling your 'pain-free' ecstatic dream are much better.

Rhythmic movement, active birth positions, breathing, relaxation, mind-quietening and distraction techniques are all necessary preparation for normal physiological birth. However, if these techniques are framed within a 'pain-free' philosophy, rather than within a philosophy that accepts the necessity of *working with* physiological pain, then the birthing woman runs the risk of having nowhere to go when it all begins to crumble.

For the willing woman, getting hung up on the idea that labour shouldn't be painful or that, with the correct technique and control, it will be painless, is, I think, a capacity-limiting viewpoint. Because what happens when it *is* painful? Then the only guaranteed pathway to that elusive 'pain-free' birth experience becomes incredibly seductive, so it's just a slippery slide to the epidural.

With these cultural attitudes to pain in general, it's no wonder it can be hard for willing women to keep a positive 'can-do' attitude to labour pain, even when they know it is healthy, functional pain.

Labour pain has received lots of bad press so certainly there's work to be done. The willing woman needs to *reframe* her understanding and relationship with pain. She needs to move past fear of pain to name it differently, to claim it, reframe it and embrace it. She needs to bypass the fear to instead read pain as potency.

Pain is power

Framing birth as a peak performance of the body, opens up a more positive take on thinking about pain in labour. Willing women undertaking the quest for normal physiological birth are challenged to work with pain—the physiological pain of their bodies working at peak levels.

In this quest pain is *power*.

This 'pain is power' metaphor works in a number of ways. Firstly, we can understand the pain—the power—as energy: birthing energy flowing through the woman's body, the energy of her body contracting, stretching, straining and opening.

Secondly, the physiological pain of labour is a catalyst for releasing birthing hormones, as I'll explain shortly—so we can think about this pain/power as the power to achieve a normal physiological birth.

Finally, 'pain is power' works in reference to pain being the pivotal point around which hierarchical institutional power oscillates; because pain and how it's handled are at the heart of the power dynamics present at birth.[40]

If the willing woman can find a way to work with the functional physiological pain of labour then this will generally enable her to stay with her intentions and maintain control over the circumstances of the birth. However, if she can't find a way to work with her pain, whoever *does* 'manage' the pain will take control of the circumstances of the birth: once pain-relief options come into play, medical considerations arise.

Let me explain this with an example. If we think of a birthing woman using an epidural to enable a pain-free birth and to 'stay in control of herself' (her behaviours and sounds) during the birth, the price she pays is a loss of power to control the circumstances of the birth. This is because the birth now becomes a medical situation. The medical practitioners around her are now the ones actively controlling the circumstances of the birth—running the drip to keep the contractions going and stabilise her blood pressure, using the catheter to empty her bladder, strapping her up to the continuous monitoring machine to keep a check on how the baby is coping with the epidural drugs, and so on. It's all now more like a patient in intensive care than a woman actively involved in a physiological process. The 'pain pathway' to the unintended cascade of interventions mentioned in chapter 2 is set in motion. By giving up her pain the birthing woman is giving up her power.

Pathological pain versus physiological pain

Because we've stuck birth in a medical frame where pain automatically becomes associated with disease and damage, most birthing women have a 'pain as a signal of danger' mindset. Or maybe, as Irma explains, we could call it an 'it's impossible!' mindset:

> Labour always seems to be characterised as something medical that is separate from and unlike anything else we have experienced in our lives, which increases the impression that it is impossible.

This is something I hear a lot. But in reality there are many aspects of the functional pain of labour that will be familiar to the willing woman. You know, if you were running around the block or oval, or going for it at a spin, pump or cardio class, or Iyengar yoga session with all your stretch receptors going to the max—what would you expect to feel in your body? Breathing changes, ragged gulping or searing breaths, lungs heaving, heart pumping, body heating, perspiring, flushing; leg muscles burning and aching, maybe even cramping—all the sensations that go with functional physical effort. Felt to a greater or lesser intensity depening on your fitness and practice levels.

So what functional effort sensations can you expect to feel in birthing? Well, you'll feel your breathing change, your heart pumping, body heating, perspiring and flushing. You'll feel all the usual effort sensations, including all those stretch receptors going to the max. After all, your body is opening to release your baby.

Think about times you've done yoga or any other form of strong stretching work. Remember that hot stretching feeling? This is the sensation I'm referring to when I talk about stretch receptors working. And there are a lot of them working during labour!

Think about stretch receptors working. They feel hot and burning when they are going to the max. They even feel as though they are tearing. These are some of the most demanding of the functional pain sensations you are going to feel in labour.

Firstly, there's the stretch of your cervix opening. Your cervix softens and opens a little when you menstruate, so you've already felt this a little bit as period pain. Of course, it opens much more to release your baby, so the sensations are definitely ramped up. Some women say they're ramped up to the power of one hundred—others to the power of infinity! Nonetheless, the cervix-opening sensations are of the same family as that period pain you may be familiar with—starting with grumbly dull heaviness, probably back ache, then crampy spikes, intensifying into the strong dragging up feeling of the cervix opening further and further. The muscle fibres that make up the cervix are being dragged up and open; the stretch receptors are hot, burning and may eventually feel like they're tearing.

Then there's a whole range of other actions occurring during labour that call on your stretch receptors:

- The ligaments anchoring your symphysis pubis and sacroiliac joints opening—stretch receptors, hot and burning, sharp and stabbing.
- The pelvis opening and spreading, pushing out into your hip joints—stretch receptors, plus hip pain and dull nerve ache down your legs.
- Pelvis opening, coccyx and sacrum pressing out to open the pelvic outlet—stretch receptors hot and burning, plus bones shifting to enable your lower back to undergo a major rearrangement.
- The baby moving down through your vagina and onto your perineum—stretch receptors hot and burning: the 'ring of fire'.

So you can see that making friends with stretch receptors is important because activated stretch receptors not only signal the opening of your body, they also trigger oxytocin and endorphin release and that sets up a feedback loop for efficient birthing.

You'll also feel rushes of hormones, causing flushing; hot and cold temperature changes; pins and needles prickling up and down your arms and through your torso; uncontrollable shaking and shivering; and possibly nausea and vomiting. You're probably quite familiar with nausea and vomiting by now, but maybe not when it's 'at the peak of a contraction' degree of difficulty.

Bowel pressure. Although the baby is in the vagina during second stage, the angle at which it's coming down through your body means it's pressing out towards the bowel. So the labouring woman will feel it as massive bowel pressure. We've all experienced bowel pressure; we all know what to do with bowel pressure—bear down and release. This is the physiological template for second stage. Yes, I know the baby doesn't come out your bum—though that's exactly what it feels like at the time! (You can imagine this is very confusing to the birthing woman.) But working with your body as if the baby were coming out your bum—bearing down and releasing—while trusting that the baby is coming out your vagina, is the labouring effort required in second stage.

Then, as well as the rush of hormones, the sensation of bowel pressure and the major challenge of burning stretch receptors, the 'overwhelm factor' is the mother of all challenges.

Many individual functionally painful sensations in labour would be manageable if they were all you were dealing with. It's just that they're all coming at you at the same time and at the same intensity—leaving you not knowing where to put your focus and then coming again and again, with hardly any break in between. That's the 'overwhelm factor' kicking in.

One of the mantras I repeat often in my workshops is 'you don't have to like it to do it brilliantly'. Another one is: 'It's only stretch receptors!'

Sounds silly? Well, a midwife told me recently she was working with one of my 'willing women' who, during the peak of the contractions was singing out, 'It's only stretch receptors, it's only stretch receptors'—worked well, apparently!

So, do you recognise some of these physical sensations you're likely to experience in labour? In recognising them do you begin to feel like they are something you could have a go at? Because if you can think of birthing as a 'peak performance of the body', alongside the other activities that you actively pursue to maintain fitness, wellbeing and to strive for personal-best achievements, you might be less likely to hold our culture's 'pain as a signal of danger' mindset in reference to birth. And you might better hold a more helpful 'pain as a signal of effort' mindset, or 'working through pain barriers' mindset.

Suffering versus potency

Maybe if birthing women connected with pain in labour as the functional physiological pain of a body working at peak performance levels then, rather than falling into the culturally reinforced 'victim to the pain' role, they could reframe pain as the functional potency of their body working at an extreme edge. And claim it, like Susan, 'as a badge of physical and spiritual strength and courage'.

The willing woman needs to weed out the deep acculturated roots of this 'victim to the pain' mentality in order to avoid the trap that will, when the labour ramps up, leave her feeling the need to be saved by all those pain-relief options. She needs to replace these negative cultural messages with positive motivation to claim the healthy functional pain of labour and embrace its intensity.

She needs to value and trust the pain in order to fire up her motivation for the work of labour. She needs to understand what's happening in her body in order to trust her body's painful signals. Then, when she feels the outrageously intense sensations of her body opening, she can go with them, breath into them. Rather than fearing and resisting them, or pulling back and fighting what her body and baby are trying to do.

She also needs to understand what's happening in her body so that her thinking, worrying brain has enough information to settle and then 'get out of the way'. This is a very important point, which I'll go into more later. Basically, her thinking brain needs to get out of the way so that her birthing instincts have half a chance of taking over the show.

Pleasures of the body working

Many of us work the pavement, the sports field, the surf, the stair master, the gym equipment, the yoga mat, the pilates 'reformer', the craggy rock face or steep incline, pushing our bodies and gritting our teeth to fulfil our resolve and claim the rewards of fitness, flexibility and exhilaration.

In fact, many of us use the 'pain is my friend' mantra to get through the inevitable pain barriers that challenge us on our fitness and achievement quests.

Many more of us undertake this physical activity for its own intrinsic reward. We take on these physically demanding and often functionally painful activities because, as well as seeking that future gain, we also relish the satisfaction in feeling the *zing* of our bodies working. We enjoy the pleasures of immediate feedback, of rhythm, muscle, heartbeat, breath. The pleasures of skill, strength, spring, and focus, all attesting to our vitality and capacity, not to mention the equally pleasurable relief that occurs after periods of intense effort.

Willing women who can reframe their relationship with functional pain can embrace the pleasures of their bodies working during labour: the satisfaction of feedback from their body opening, the relief between contractions, the achievement gained, contraction by contraction.

Emotional and psychological pain

Generally we think about pain in childbirth as physical, and of course there's a hell of a lot going on physically, so it's understandable that we can become fixated on that. But that's only part of it because there's a whole psycho-emotional pain dimension to birth as well. In reality all pain is multidimensional. There is the physical or sensory dimension; there is the emotional dimension; there is the thinking dimension (coping thinking or distress thinking); there is the environmental dimension that can raise or lower our pain tolerance making any pain seem more or less intense; and there is the pain behaviours dimension (the patterns of expected pain behaviours influenced by our families or our culture).

For many women, in fact, childbirth activates *layers* of pain. Women often give expression to 'the pain of ages'. This is the pain of womankind, the pain passed through their generational line (their mothers and grandmothers) and also to their own personal emotional pain arising perhaps from their own birth, their childhood and life experiences. Or it may arise from their present reality or stem from fears projected into the future.

In labour a woman may become a vessel for all this pain—cultural, gendered, generational and personal, as Nancy found:

> But it's with the psychological and emotional stuff—that's where I feel I have to call my support in. I need people to assist me with positive pathways in my brain, not going into my mother's or my grandmother's old fears. It's to support me around that stuff, not the physical work of birthing.

Transforming psychological pain is powerful work. And birthing women supported to be in the full potency of the alchemical transformation of pain into power, are certainly initiated as powerful mothers.

Pain as the pathway to your birth-friendly hormones

Oxytocin, plus endorphins, plus adrenalin: this is the simple version of the basic hormonal formula for normal physiological birth. And functional pain is one of the catalytic agents for this hormonal mix.

We need high levels of oxytocin to drive the contractions; these contractions create functional physiological pain, which causes the release of endorphins. The endorphins give some moderation of the pain, but more importantly they swamp the 'thinking brain' to release the labouring woman's birthing instincts. Then there are two important surges of adrenalin at particular points in the labour—right when they're most needed.

It's an amazingly tailored recipe, refined over the ages. And embracing and working with the normal functional pain of labour is a key to unlocking this hormonal formula.

Oxytocin

Oxytocin is often called the 'tend and befriend' hormone, the 'calm and connect' hormone, the 'luurve' hormone. It's a neurotransmitter that influences many body systems and behaviours. It stems from our mammalian heritage and is involved in all our sweet connections—from soothing and calming, all the way through to our sexual responsiveness and orgasmic release, as well as bonding with our babies, partners, family and friends.[41] Or, as one midwife says, 'it is simply a big injection of instinctive love'. You're 'oxytocinised' anytime you get that sweet connected buzz, that 'lovingness' experience. Bring it on!

In birthing, oxytocin has an extra role. It is released in regular pulses that increase in frequency through the labour and drive the contractions—the muscular waves that facilitate the opening of your body and the release of your baby.

Even while being the driver of those big powerful contractions though, oxytocin does not leave us without resources. Oxytocin raises our pain tolerance, both through integration with the endorphin system and also because the connected buzz and 'lovingness vibe' it creates draws in soothing and nurturing human support.

Oxytocin is one of the hormones that drive humans to be social, cooperative beings. These oxytocin states are catching—oxytocin has a pheromonal effect, so as well as pulsing in our bodies it's also secreted—so let's hope the birthing space is pumping with an oxytocin 'lovingness' vibe to support the birthing woman's hormonal surges and to help everyone fall well and truly in love with the baby.

Endorphins

These are our natural opiates—the 'feel-good' hormones. You can get some from chocolate and good experiences but we get more of them during high-intensity physical activity that involves functional physiological pain.

Endorphins take the edge off the pain and bring on a 'runner's high'. Surely you want to experience the equivalent 'birther's high'? But even more important than this high, as far as normal physiological birthing goes, is the way endorphins 'take out' the cerebral cortex (the judging, thinking, planning brain). They bring on a trance-like state and reduce our inhibitions, setting off a shift in consciousness that triggers what I refer to as 'the evolutionary regression'. I'll expand on this vital concept later in the chapter, but for now you'll have a sense of what I'm referring to if I say this shift of consciousness releases 'primal woman' (or what midwife Ina May Gaskin calls our 'monkey')[42] loose to get on with birthing.

When birthing women are beautifully 'endorphined' they look tired, exhausted, completely out of it or 'on the nod' (or 'labour drunk' as one mother named it) which can be both confusing and concerning to the inexperienced. If you didn't know differently you would be sucked into believing that the birthing woman is exhausted and can't possibly go on. The woman herself feels the effect of this surge of endorphins as tiredness and exhaustion, of being out of it—and if she has been up all night then that will lend weight to this interpretation of tiredness.

But I have to tell you that when these endorphins hit, all birthing women look the same. They look and feel exhausted in the same way, regardless of whether they've been going at their labour for a few days or only an hour or so after a full night's sleep. So *feeling* exhausted and actually *being* physiologically exhausted are two different things. Occasionally, exhaustion might really be part of the picture, but this will show up as physiological markers (such as pulse and dehydration markers) not just as looking and feeling exhausted.

Trust this 'endorphined' feeling. It's opening the way to your instincts.

Now, to complete the basic hormonal formula for normal physiological birthing, some shots of adrenalin get thrown in.

Adrenalin

Adrenalin is known as the 'fight or flight' hormone. It's produced when we are on high alert, feel threatened, fearful, anxious or angry. At low levels it primes us for action, while high levels trigger our primal survival defence systems—fight, flight or freeze.

Ideally, there are only two key surges of adrenalin during birthing—both necessary to prime us for action in labour. The first marks early labour and primes you for the action to come. Another in second stage awakens you from the 'on the nod' experience of the endorphins and primes you for the birth of your baby.

However, if there is ongoing adrenalin release, this will not be helpful. If a birthing woman becomes highly adrenalised and is not able to be soothed, then her labour will be compromised. In fact, this will cause the labour to be more painful, too slow, or to stall completely.

Remember, too, that adrenalised states are catching. And if the birth space becomes adrenalised that's not going to be great for the birth.

Hopefully you can see the way in which our natural birth hormones create a wonderful feedback loop—high oxytocin leads to strong contractions, leads to functional pain, leads to endorphin release, leads to our instinctive capacity taking over, leads to further surges of oxytocin, leads to stronger contractions, and on and on. Yes, that's the loop for efficient birthing. All you have to do is find a way to work with the pain to set this loop in motion.

Stages of labour and hormonal surges (Fig 3.1)

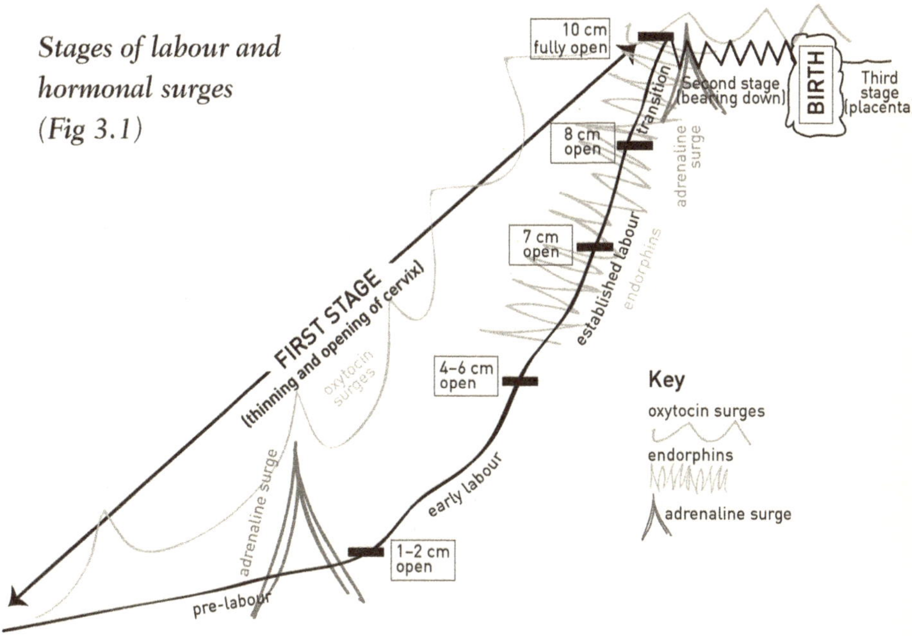

Hormones and sexuality

Before we go on to talk more about instincts I want to add another word or two about hormones, primal woman, birthing and sexuality. To do this we need to take a wider view of sexuality and see it as a part of the expressive energy of life. Because let me tell you that birth and sex have a lot in common.

Both share aspects of the same hormonal formula, the same body parts, the same surrender to our body's lead, and the same building rhythms—contractions arising, peaking, ebbing away only to arise again, over and over. The entire birth fits within an orgasmic pattern: energy arising, building intensity, peaking, expressing, releasing then softening into the after-glow.

And both birthing and sex share the same requirements for comfortable adaptable furnishings, room to move, mood lighting, warmth—unless you're turned on by bright lights, cold sterile surroundings, being confined to a narrow, high, uncomfortable bed, and attached to surveillance machines with strangers coming in and out observing and commenting on your timing and progress! No? That doesn't get you going? Well then, think about the kind of atmosphere that might set the mood for birthing—one with intimacy, trust and privacy.

Maybe you can't get your head around putting sexual responsiveness and birth in the same basket. After all, the passionate, uninhibited, sexy free spirit so encouraged (if not demanded) as a present-day aspiration for women can be placed under great strain during pregnancy, birth and early mothering. However, in normal physiological birthing there is a wonderful opportunity for harmonising these aspects of ourselves.

When women embrace the intensity of birth and surrender to the hormonally orchestrated passions of birthing energy; when they give themselves uninhibitedly to the strong demands of the labour, finding their 'birth song' and 'birth dance' and flowing with the building intensity and the orgasmic rhythm—its peaking and releasing, contraction after contraction—until ecstatically releasing their babies with that love bomb of hormones, then they may have a new experience of their innate sexuality.

Instinctive birthing: surrendering to the evolutionary regression

What I refer to as the evolutionary regression goes hand in hand with normal physiological birthing.

We have been birthing ourselves generation by generation across our human history since before we developed our cerebral cortex. Now, don't get me wrong—our cerebral cortex is very impressive across so much of our lives, but it's really not helpful at all when it comes to our birthing capacity. In fact, it's a liability, and the sooner it gets taken out of the picture, the better for the birth!

This is exactly what happens during the evolutionary regression, thanks to the birth hormones. When those surges of hormones really get going, they not only drive the contractions but also bring on the drifty state of altered consciousness that is so necessary in triggering this evolutionary regression. When this regression happens, twenty-first-century latte-sipping chic dissolves and the primal birthing woman emerges.

The hormones get this process going. However, the ease with which the regression unfolds will also have to do with your ability to drop out of your 'thinking', 'controlling', 'judging' brain to become spontaneous and uninhibited (hopefully without relying on alcohol!). Because becoming uninhibited in labour is the forerunner to instinctive expression—the forerunner to unleashing 'primal woman'.

Getting to know your instincts

Have you, like Jacinta, made friends with 'primal woman' somewhere in your life? Jacinta says:

> I know primal woman; I have met her and I love her and I love to let her take me over. I know how important she is and I have tried to cultivate her and let her brim out of me, wild.

Getting friendly with her is task number one for willing women, so that you can trust her and respond to her instinctive urges in labour. Yael says:

> All that breathing and groaning that my primal self did was perfect, I imagined each of those strong contractions moving the baby down. After about three hours of real intense labour, feeling like I was completely stoned, I had about half an hour bearing down and then our gorgeous baby popped out.

It's not so easy to trust primal woman though if you have been keeping her on a tight leash all your adult life.

Many success strategies for contemporary women to find a place of achievement in the world, are based on male-patterned, rational right-brained thinking or gender-neutral pathways which require control of their reproductive bodies, their menstruating, pregnant, birthing or lactating bodies and denial of their emotional, intuitive, instinctive selves. These controlling tendencies can work against women though when it comes to normal physiological birthing, because many women continue in control mode, rather than softening, trusting and following their body's lead and surrendering to its instinctive rhythms.

Some women are already well practised at being in tune with instinctive primal woman. Their lifestyles support an instinctive approach that gives them not only a trust in their instinctive nature but also a lived experience of following their instincts.

Many of us, on the other hand, wouldn't know an instinct if we fell over it. Because, as author and psychotherapist Stephanie Dowrick says, 'When our instincts nudge us, many of us routinely override them'.[43]

Our instinctive nature is expressed through our capacity to follow our body signals. The signals that prompt us to eat and drink when hungry and thirsty; to discern what is healthy, rather than what is influenced by emotional need, convenience or TV ads; to follow our evacuative instincts when they call, rather than habitually controlling them because of social or work constraints or lack of access to a clean toilet; to balance activity and rest periods according to our body's instinctive need rather than because it's too cold or wet or we're too tired (or insert your excuse here).

To be in touch with our body signals is to sleep and rise according to our body clock rather than the work clock, the study clock, the TV clock, the internet clock or any other of the many clocks that can direct our days and nights. It is to give expression to our innate needs for intimacy, sensuality and sexuality through surrender to our body impulses. In short, we need to allow our instinctive needs at least some influence over our daily rhythms, rather than controlling our instinctive nature entirely out of existence.

In my workshops I ask women to reflect on how often they are guided by their body instincts and how often they override them. By doing the same, you can gain some idea of how practised you are at following your body instincts. How often do you go to sleep when you're tired instead of being directed by what time it is? How often do you go to the toilet because your body needs to, instead of waiting until you are on a break at work?

Of course, reining in our instinctive drives does also have a place. However, to over-control them to the point of being unable to discern our instinctive urges is not without its negative consequences to our health and wellbeing and particularly to our birthing capacity.

Hopefully, a willing woman has a robust connection to her body instincts, but even if she does it's still not easy to connect with *birthing* instincts. As we've discussed earlier, a birthing woman will face a thick fog of pain signals, and these can certainly wreak havoc with her ability to tune in to those birthing instincts.

Having someone with her (generally an experienced woman) who can 'stand in' for her instincts, someone who can interpret and amplify the birthing instincts and guide the birthing woman to follow them through that fog of pain signals—that's the antidote for a woman struggling to connect to her birthing instincts.

Please note though that this surrendering to birthing instincts—to the primal sounds and movements emerging spontaneously during birth—should not be confused with the panicky distressed screaming of unsupported birthing women being overwhelmed by pain instincts and struggling in a negative, fearful 'pain lock'. Let me explain.

Birthing instincts versus pain instincts

Being able to tell the difference between powerful, straining, functionally painful 'effort' responses and painful *resistance* responses, is important body awareness.

In a birthing context, this means a capacity to read in the body the difference between behaviours that arise from birthing instincts, and the behaviours that arise from pain-avoiding instincts.

Birthing instincts arise from first receiving sensations coming from the body—ligaments, joints and bones shifting and spreading, changes in muscle movement, contraction and relaxation pressures, stretch receptors going to the max, posture changes, baby kicking, nuzzling, pushing and rotating. Birthing instincts awaken in response to these sensations. To follow them, willing women need to be able to accommodate these strong body sensations rather than resist them.

Birthing instincts, if they are followed spontaneously, would see birthing women releasing and opening their bodies; loosening muscles, joints, sphincter, pelvis, knees, buttocks, cervix, vagina, perineum—letting go in a free flow of open, active, instinctive movements.

On the other hand, pain-avoidance instincts, the instinctive defensive reflexes that are our survival necessities, cause our bodies to tighten and close in protective stances, or tense and pull away from painful stimuli. Think of the way we react when we touch something burning hot. Of course, these instincts are helpful if a pain stimulus is coming from outside our body and is a danger to us. But what happens when the pain arises from within our bodies and, far from being a danger to us, is rather a powerful expression of our body working? What to do with our pain-avoiding instincts then?

Birthing women taken over by their pain-avoidance instincts close up and pull away, resisting, tensing, tightening, bracing and fighting against the internal opening that the body is trying to accomplish. This 'fighting against' only makes matters worse both in terms of the pain and the progress of the labour, particularly if birthing women, on top of any internal resistance, already have the free flow of their instinctive birthing movements restricted by imposed positions (such as being confined to a narrow bed, tethered by drips, wires, belts and electrodes or strapped up in stirrups).

In a birthing context—or yoga, or an aerobics session, a pump or spin class or a training run, or any other situation where we might experience functional effort-filled pain and hit a pain barrier—how do we accommodate the functional pain and stay with our body's straining effort? How do we stay with it rather than resisting and tightening in response to our pain-avoiding instincts?

Being able to tell the difference between our body's working efforts and our pain-avoiding instincts is part of it. Being familiar with ways to raise your pain tolerance—the use of rhythm, movement and breath to work into functional pain and effort—is another. Having an intention to continue on, and finally, having facilitating support, are other means of overcoming our pain-avoidance instincts.

This is where a birthing woman's support circle, set up to support her birthing capacity, can make the greatest difference. Which instincts are going to prevail? Her birthing instincts or her pain-avoiding instincts? Which instincts are going to be amplified by her support circle? Will it be her 'Yes I can', or her 'No I can't'?

Ideally, the willing woman will be surrounded by caregivers and support people who can read these differences in her body and who can, if the need arises, call her past her resistance, and into the full and free expression of her birthing instincts.

What we are talking about here is coming up against and working through pain barriers and our pain-tolerance thresholds.

It's tricky for the birthing woman because the more she opens up to and works with her birthing instincts, the stronger the functional pain becomes—because a beautifully progressing labour is continually upping the ante. Breath by breath across her contractions, she can be on an edge between releasing into it or pulling away from it. As she surrenders to her birthing instincts the functional pain of her body working intensifies, which then means a pain-avoiding impulse to pull back can overcome her.

It's a demanding edge, often expressed as it was by Krissy when she called out across her contractions:

> I can't. Oh, no, no; oh, yes, yes I can, no, no, yes, yes, I can, I can, come on. Can I? No, no, yes, yes I can.

Melissa too expressed this edge when the intensity of her labour started to build. She found herself thinking:

> 'No, no, no' and shaking my head during contractions. As soon as I became aware of it, I consciously committed to welcoming the contractions and the pain, and so started nodding and saying, 'yes, yes, yes'.

For many labouring women this struggle between birthing instincts and pain instincts becomes a moment-by-moment tussle that can go either way, depending on the support she receives.

Joanne's story

Joanne describes just such a struggle and the way we worked through it together:

> I was feeling ready to push but I was not going ahead. I was stopping it by squeezing my buttocks together, which I had been doing for half an hour or so. I was at a mental block, fighting it. I kept saying 'it's coming, it's coming', but I wouldn't let it out. I was really scared and I couldn't focus on anything. I was in a state of 'nowhere' confusion, my mind couldn't focus on anything as I was being swept away with the pain.
>
> Rhea suggested that I spend some time on the toilet. I kept saying 'I can't move'. 'No.' 'I can't.' Then Mark whispered to me, 'Listen to Rhea, you trust her don't you?' So both Mark and Rhea practically carried me to the toilet in between powerful contractions. I had one contraction on the toilet and I still said 'I can't'. Rhea said to me with a reassuring gaze, 'Let's focus on sitting into the contraction and release into that bearing down'. So I pushed and focused and the membranes began to show. Things got moving so I moved back to the bed, leaning over the beanbag on top of the bed.
>
> I got scared again as the pain was unbearable. 'No, no, I can't.' I reached physically and emotionally for Rhea. She kept

> saying, 'Good, good, this will be a lunch-time baby', very calmly. She encouraged me to feel inside to try and feel the baby's head—this was a great focusing action to take—and my darling girl was so close, just waiting in there, and she was born before lunch!

A mother who is working with her birthing instincts will be active and spontaneous with wide-stance, free-flowing, rhythmic primal movements—rocking, swaying, stamping, stretching, embracing, bending, descending, squatting—dancing out the steps that allow her to open her body to make space for her baby to emerge.

As well as surrendering to her birth dance, the woman in touch with her birthing instincts will also freely sing out her birth song, her natural response to the physical effort, just like Kari:

> Every contraction had a voice. I moaned, I yelled, I howled. I heard the sounds as if they were outside my body, so powerful—the sounds of something wild and raw.

And Deb:

> I found the rhythm of my birth dance, freeing up—now I was working with it rather than against it. I was very vocal but this enabled me to endure the pain of each contraction.

However, the mother overtaken by fear or pain-avoidance instincts will resist and tense—not only her body against its own efforts to open: she will restrict her breath and strain her voice in high, tight, panic sounds, becoming more and more distraught. Says Vicki:

> My contractions were so full on and I was really fighting them instead of giving into them, screaming and hardly breathing.

'Calm and in control' issue

Surrendering to birthing instincts can be a very frightening proposition for some women. And not necessarily because they are afraid of the pain. Instead, some women are concerned about how they will behave in *reaction* to the pain.

Many women are therefore motivated to pursue pain-avoiding pathways because they want to 'stay calm and in control of themselves'. Perhaps the idea of being calm and in control sounds reasonable to you, but if you want to optimise your birth hormones, it's not necessarily what you want to be aiming for.

If a woman's motivation is to 'be in control' (and I'm referring here to being in control of herself, rather than the idea of controlling the circumstances of her birth, through choice of caregivers and birth place), this is often a wish to remain 'ego' or 'I'-focused. To stay in control of her behaviours and sounds, to stay 'nice', rather than freeing primal woman and allowing the evolutionary regression described earlier to do its best work. That is, her wish is to remain in the realm of the cerebral cortex—the judging, thinking, planning, controlling brain. This is what we might call 'staying in your head'. Again, you might think this sounds reasonable, but staying in your head is incredibly problematic because your cerebral cortex knows *fuck all* about birthing.

This desire to stay in your head, to stay 'in control', is a motivation for some women to seek out those pain-free-promising birth preparation techniques. They're not only motivated by fear of the pain but also by this fear of 'losing control', 'losing their dignity' and then feeling shamed or embarrassed about their behaviour.

Coming from a realistic place in regards to functional pain and using any birth skills and relaxation techniques as a way to expand your skill set for *working with pain*, that's fine. But if your choice of such techniques is driven by fear, pain-avoidance, or this desire to stay 'in control', that's a different matter.

If you are a willing woman then developing skills in breathing, relaxation, active positions and pain-tolerance techniques in preparation for working with the functional pain of labour, rather than seeking a 'pain-free' birth, would be a better fit with your expectations of normal physiological childbirth.

Embracing the intensity of the functional pain of your body working; surrendering to the 'shift in consciousness' brought about by the endorphins flooding the cerebral cortex; allowing these endorphins to help the primitive brain take over the show and prompt your instinctive birth song and dance—this is the way to go for normal physiological birthing.

Besides, if your birth does happen to be less painful than you expect, it's far easier to adjust to that than to find that your naïve expectations of 'in control', pain-free birthing have crashed on the rocks of early or established labour. Where to then?

For many women today, it's straight to the epidural—the big daddy of the 'staying in control' tool kit.

The seduction of the epidural

The seduction of the epidural is now so deeply etched into the psyche of the contemporary birthing woman that in the sporting vernacular its popularity has not only shifted the goal posts but changed the entire bloody playing field of birth.

Every birthing woman and her birth team, including the savvy 'willing' women, know that an epidural is just outside the birth room door, holding out the promise of a pain-free comfortable birth as well as the possibility of the birthing woman 'staying in control of herself'.

The rise and rise of the epidural has broadsided the various movements that, over the past few decades, have championed the benefits of normal physiological birth. Gone now is the need for relaxation skills, gone is the need for directed breathing, gone is the need for active positions for women to work with their bodies and babies. Gone is the need for the enriching experience of deeply connected human support; gone is the need for the personal growth required in order for birthing women to access their personal agency; gone are the normal physiological hormonal surges. And gone too is the possibility of surrendering to the 'shift in consciousness' brought on by hormones that allows a taste of the expansive, creative mystery lying beyond our everyday consciousness.

In my early years of birth work, when women reached any distress point in their labour, the birthing woman's familiar pleading would be expressed in the lament of 'help me, help me'. Of course, if you think about it, this request offers the support team some room to manoeuvre and many support possibilities to work with. We can 'help' with encouragement, massage, movement, heat, water, changing positions or people or place or energy. The list goes on. In this present labour-bypass era though, the seduction of the epidural has reshaped the nature of support dynamics, both in expectations and in practice. The pleading for 'help' has now become the *demand* for an epidural, making it much harder for a support team to manoeuvre around the command to *get me the fucking epidural now!*

And I don't care what she says before the labour about 'hating needles' and that she 'definitely won't be having any epidural'. This is a naïve defence against the seductive pull of the epidural. Because when it comes to a 'pain panic' in labour, a woman's fear of needles, or catheters, or drips and medical technology will appear trivial, dissolving in comparison to the allure of being pain free in this panic moment. And given that recent research in neuroscience is proving that emotions are the most powerful drivers of our decision-making, what's going to happen next is a no-brainer.

At a long, tiring first birth some years ago I heard the epidural's seductive song whispering in my own ears. I found myself musing on how good it would be if the birthing woman had an epidural so we could *all* get some sleep! It shocked me, so after that birth (which did eventually unfold normally without the epidural) I decided that I needed to undertake something in my own life that would put me back in touch with stamina, effort and functional pain realities. Taking up marathon kayaking seemed the obvious answer and has certainly put me back in touch with pain barriers and crisis points!

I can certainly give you a vivid description of my predictable crisis points in a 22 km marathon paddle. At around 17 km, when I'm seriously being 'asked the question', the safety boat (the marathon kayaking equivalent of an epidural) is seductively tempting. This is when I find myself thinking 'maybe I could just "accidentally" fall out and get picked up in the tinnie and taken to the finish line for a hot cuppa'—thoughts that need to be shouted down as I dig deep into my resolve, stamina, rhythm and stroke techniques.

How does the 'epidural seduction effect' manifest in any of your challenging pursuits?

Pain threshold and pain-tolerance levels

Many of us think of our pain threshold as something set at a particular immovable point—that we either have a low pain threshold or a high pain threshold and nothing will change that. But this is not the case.

Most of us register painful stimuli such as electric shocks at a similar point (don't ask me about how they did that research!), but that's not the same as your pain threshold or, more importantly, your pain-tolerance level. Pain-tolerance levels vary from person to person and also over time. Your pain-tolerance level can be raised or lowered by many factors. The willing woman needs to understand what will work for her to raise her pain tolerance. Also, hopefully, her partner and support team have insight into how to boost her pain-tolerance levels.

Comfort zone to transformation zone

Many of us live our lives understanding the importance of expanding our comfort zone, being on a growing edge, a learning edge. As child psychiatrist Bruce Perry explains: 'Each of us has a comfort zone in which we feel totally safe. In this zone, we aren't learning much because anything even a little bit new will cause a tiny dose of stress.'[44]

We all have our comfort zones—our physical, emotional, psychological, social, relational and other comfort zones. Those of us who regularly take on challenges that keep us on a 'growth edge' are well practised at expanding our comfort zone through pushing the edges of our discomfort and pain zones. Flow theory, which I mentioned in chapter 1, is premised on being on these growth edges.

The following reflective tool can be a useful way of thinking about being on a growth edge in any challenging aspects of life.

Think about three concentric circles. The inner circle represents your *comfort zone*, the next circle represents your *discomfort zone* and the outer circle represents your *pain zone*. There is a fourth circle, which I describe as representing a *transformation zone*, which we'll come to later. For now let's stay with the three circles.

Zones (Fig 3.2)

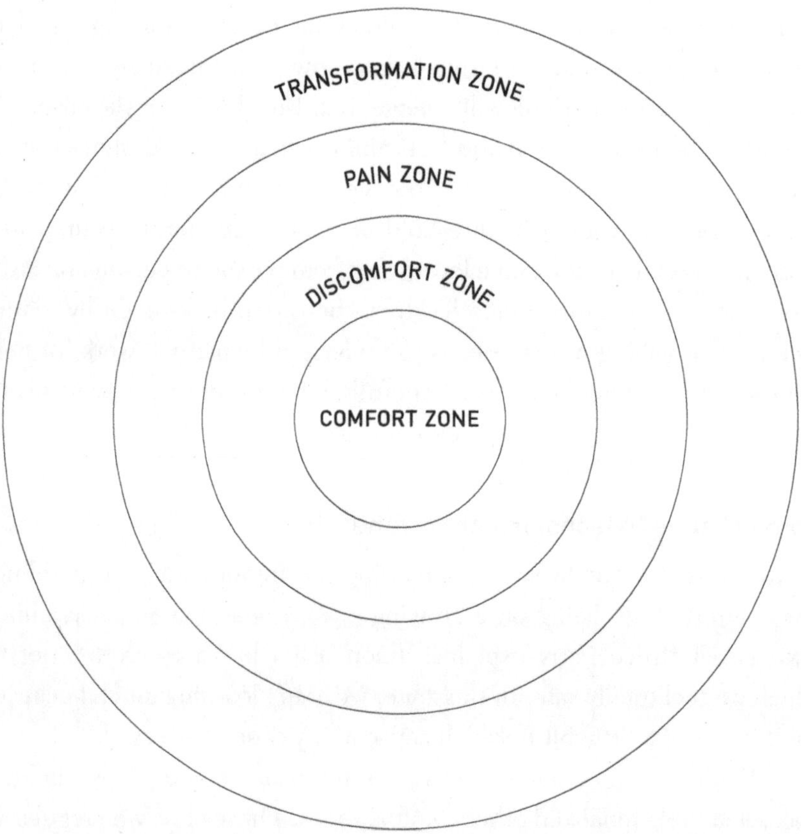

To begin picturing these zones, just imagine if you had to walk up a long, steep incline. Would that fall within your physical comfort zone? What about if you had to sprint up that steep incline, would that take you into your physical discomfort zone or even your pain zone? Would sprinting up that same incline while carrying a heavy backpack take you out of your discomfort zone and drag you well into your pain zone?

Or maybe you can engage with the idea of moving through these zones if you imagine some public-speaking scenarios. Maybe speaking in front of your family and friends is within your emotional comfort zone, while speaking to your work colleagues would take you into an emotional discomfort zone—and speaking in front of strangers would really ramp up your emotional pain and spin you into your pain zone.

Let's apply these circles to birthing. Ideally, willing women will, through previous experiences of working with their healthy striving bodies, have gained an expanded comfort zone. Additionally, these experiences with their bodies will also have enabled them to normalise working in a *discomfort* zone, which in turn will push out the edge before she reaches her *pain* zone.

Then, by having a normalising attitude to painful functional physiological demands on her body, as well as a habituating practice of 'working with pain' skills (breathing, releasing, birth positions, etc.), and boosted by experienced support for working with pain, she will also be well set up to expand her capacity to work in her pain zone.

As Nancy explains:

> As a dancer and physical performer I enjoy the physical. So, because I had experienced physiological pain so many times, I was naïve and said, 'Oh yes, I want to experience that in birth'. But when some of those contractions really kicked in and were really painful I suddenly did get a bit freaked out and needed support to trust that and work into that next level of intensity.

The aim, of course, is to be able to expand your comfort zone to include what previously had been a discomfort zone, thereby pushing out the 'edges' of these zones to give more breathing space before hitting a pain zone.

Then, the aim is to increase your tolerance for working in a pain zone, thereby pushing out the edge to the transformation zone. Let's continue with the 'sprinting up steep inclines' scenario here. If you were training and running more, you would expand your comfort zone, not only because of fitness but also because of building up your pain tolerance. This would enable you to take on more and more steep inclines, even with a backpack, before you were into your discomfort zone or eventually your pain zone. If you kept going up and over those rises and came racing down the descent on the other side, you would move out of your pain zone and experience that 'runner's high', taking you way out into a *transformation* zone.

It's at the 'edges' of these zones that what might be called pain barriers come up; barriers that, unless normalised and supported, can blow out into a 'crisis of confidence'—that feeling that you can't go on and you want to give up.

A woman's familiarity with moving through these zones; her self-awareness about what helps or hinders her capacity to adjust as she hits these edges and moves through these zones; her acceptance that birthing will call upon her to move through them, and her willingness to go on that challenging ride—all will have an impact on her pain-tolerance levels.

Some of us have the body memory of stamina from experiences of our bodies working hard to achieve a physical goal. Others of us may also have a memory of mental and emotional stamina because of experiences of focused, disciplined application to achieve goals in education, work or other demanding mental pursuits, or because of life circumstances that have expanded our emotional stamina.

Whatever the case, if we have felt the rewards of once stretching our stamina and endurance—our 'growing edge'—physical or otherwise, then this experience provides the bedrock of our capacity for endurance and transformation in birthing.

Finally, hopefully, as the birthing woman surrenders to this intensifying process and her hormones facilitate the evolutionary regression that allows her instincts to kick in, she passes through the pain zone and on into the fourth circle, the transformation zone.

Transformation zone

One of the opportunities given by birthing is this potential for transcendent shifts in consciousness and transformation. Mali says:

> With each contraction there was pain, but to say it 'hurt' would be inaccurate, or at least incomplete.
>
> 'Pain' is perhaps a workable euphemism for the indefinable; really it was an unequalled, inescapable intensity, just teetering on the edge of bearable. An experience of being utterly, irrevocably bound to the body but, at the same time, privy to those transcendent dimensions of self that were hereunto inaccessible, even unknown to me before this moment. Unlike any other pain that I had previously endured, this pain I journeyed—and so embraced my passion and courage and power on the way.

As Mali's experience suggests, pain is the potent catalyst for transcendent and transformative experiences in birthing. If a birthing woman is supported to trust and work with the pain, to surrender to the hormonal processes, she will be enabled to transcend her ego, her rational control mechanisms and transcend her previously known capacity in order to reveal new and deeper resources for mothering.

Building pain tolerance

Tamara's observations about the parallels between dance and birthing, I think, get to the heart of the matter of extending comfort zones and building pain tolerance:

> As a dancer, my primary source of identity has been with my body, experienced as powerful, strong, capable, willing, obedient,

> natural, working, and a conduit to transcendent experience through movement. When I view birth through the lens of 'body' I can absolutely understand the state of 'suspended mind/working body' that is so necessary to facilitate an instinctual normal physiological childbirth. Dance in performance leaves the cerebral cortex, the thinking brain, at the door, and relies on the memory of trained muscles to act almost without direction …

Willing women, especially those whose lifestyle has not served them in building up habituated 'working with pain' skills (a habit of slowing and deepening your breathing, a habit of relaxing your muscles, a habit of rhythmic movement) will need, perhaps like a dancer, to practise to the point of habituation the active birth positions and strategies that will provide a springboard for instinctive birthing behaviours and the 'evolutionary regression' to kick in.

Building up a familiarity with these movements will enable the willing woman to more readily surrender to her birthing instincts, instead of being hijacked by her pain instincts. The idea of this 'practise till habituation' is not about 'control over' but rather a 'path in' and is the foundation to surrendering to your birthing instincts.

Some women might think, 'Oh, well, if it's instinctive I don't need education or practice, I'll just know what to do'. Well, if you still have a strong family or cultural connection to, and trust of, normal physiological birth alive in your muscle memory and psyche, that might be true. But most of us will need enough information to settle our cerebral cortex and enough body experiences of physiological effort and movement to trust and surrender, even through that fog of functional pain in labour.

So as well as backing her intentions by making wise birth choices, the willing woman does have active physical preparation to do. She needs to develop a practised and habituated skill set for building her pain tolerance and 'working with pain'—breath work, body work, release and relaxation practices, stamina-building work, yoga, swimming, walking, dancing, and active birth practice to adopt the open-pelvis positions and movements necessary for birthing.

Boosting pain tolerance in the labour-bypass era

Okay, so you're a willing woman, or at least a tentative willing woman. You've got your values and motivation sorted, you've reframed your attitude to pain, you're prepared to give primal woman an airing and you're excited about the orgasmic bit. Great!

Unfortunately, it's still not easy. Because remember, you are birthing in the labour-bypass era. How will this affect your pain tolerance?

Birth space

When people come into your home, how do you want them to feel? Welcome? Relaxed? Does the way you have so carefully set up your space invite them in?

Many of us pay particular attention to the unspoken messages given by our living spaces. We guide expectations of behaviour, activity and mood through placement of furniture, use of lighting, visual delights and soundscapes. Even if you don't put much thought into these things they nonetheless influence us all subliminally. After all, we don't spend a fortune on architects, interior designers and landscape specialists for nothing.

Architects and interior designers study the power of the placement of material objects in relation to each other, to direct movement, behaviour, expectation and feelings. Sometimes it's overt, other times it's subtle, so that when we come into any new space we are taking in both direct and implied cues about behaviour and expectations.

In birthing spaces, where the narrow whizz-bang hospital bed, electronic equipment, bright lights and sterile instruments dominate, the message is very clear—'you're in a workplace, where medical stuff is going to happen, so get up on the bed and do as you are told!'

It's interesting to note that in the UK, as reported in 'Normalising Birth in England: a qualitative study', in hospital settings proactive for normal birth, 'clinical guidelines indicated that women should be kept out of bed if possible. Beds were kept in the highest position possible and midwives spread their charting on it, so it was literally difficult to access.'[45]

Going into hospital labour rooms, I'm always struck by how cold and stark they are. Nothing to distract, to soften, to warm, to please the eye and soothe the feelings; nothing giving either implied or direct messages to move freely, to be spontaneous, to trust the physiological process; nothing to boost oxytocin and endorphin release.

Our birthing rooms are not set up to back you in your quest for normal physiological birth. These rooms are set up for access to medical equipment. They are set up in response to institutional requirements—cleaning, occupational health and safety, standardisation, electronic surveillance and record keeping. (Now I know computers are a wonderful addition to our lives, but trust me, having them in the birth space is the last thing you need if you are trying to access primal woman!)

The idea of 'birth space', which includes the physical environment as well as the power dynamics at play within the birth space, has been researched and critiqued by academics around the world. Over the past few years in Australia these ideas have been expressed in the concept of 'Birth Territory', as outlined in the book *Birth Territory and Midwifery Guardianship*.[46] According to this concept, such medicalised birth rooms are defined as 'surveillance rooms'. A surveillance room, as described by Professor of Midwifery Kathleen Fahy in the book, 'denotes a clinical environment designed to facilitate surveillance of the woman and to optimise the ease and comfort of the staff'.

In contrast to a surveillance room, *Birth Territory* also describes a 'sanctum' as 'a homely environment designed to optimise the privacy, ease and comfort of the woman, to optimise physiological function and emotional wellbeing'. These sanctum birth spaces have access to all that medical equipment but it's hidden away, not in your face dictating your actions.

Willing women and their support teams need to be on the case about this. They need to create a 'sanctum' within the confines of the standard 'surveillance room'. They need to override institutional and medicalised messages and claim the space for the work of physiological birthing and for building that loving feeling that will 'oxytocinise' the birth space.

They need to protect the space to achieve the privacy necessary for optimising birth hormones and birthing instincts; create an environment that will raise their pain-tolerance levels; support the needed mixture of soothed feelings and physical invigoration. They need to honour the birth space as a personal intimate space, a sacred space that facilitates an inward focus and a woman's ability to be attuned to her baby.

Move the bed, make space for working with your labour—for pacing, rocking, leaning, bouncing and rotating on the ball, creating a burying nest. Dim the lights for spontaneity; add softness, warmth, beauty, positive distractions, familiar things, uplifting things, music to orchestrate the energy—lifting it, settling it, sustaining it, changing it. Put obstacles between you and the door to create the nesting cave-like privacy needed for primal woman to emerge.

Hopefully you can also access nature or a garden to soothe, to distract, to inspire. I'm reminded of the many productive birthing hours I've previously spent with women pacing around the Fitzroy Gardens in Melbourne when one of our major public hospitals was situated adjacent to this park. Finding a tree to hang off or lean into for support, being distracted by counting possums at night, enjoying the pleasure of wind, sun, moon, stars—all wonderful support for raising pain tolerance.

But I'm also reminded of the more usual situation of women labouring in rooms with no view, let alone any access—even by being able to open a window—to fresh air or outdoors.

When women create their own birth space it's very different. There are female architects who have studied the spontaneous movements of birthing women and translated this into the design of birth rooms that follow these movements.[47] Women birthing at home can, of course, create a personalised, inspiring birth space incorporating indoor and outdoor nests and sanctuaries to raise their pain thresholds and to maximise their birthing capacity.

Then, of course, there is the essential element of access to water—at least a shower, but more especially a birth tub. Separate to the issue of water birth (birthing the baby into the water), the availability of water immersion for labouring is so beneficial for hormonal release, boosting your pain tolerance and facilitating normal physiological birthing. No willing woman should be without it!

Diminishing pain tolerance

Now I want to talk about some of the things that can diminish a birthing woman's pain tolerance. And first off, I would have to say that just about everything that a birthing woman will encounter in a typical hospital setting during her labour will, by default, have the unintended consequence of diminishing her pain tolerance—the physical setting, the procedures and interruptions that disturb her rhythm, the questions and discussions that require the engagement of her cerebral cortex. The list goes on and on.

I can't tell you how many times I've seen birthing women surrendering to the evolutionary regression and watched the labour going so wonderfully, only to have it all hijacked when she gets to the hospital and somebody starts asking her questions about the date of her last menstrual period or the dates of her scans—all requiring high-end cerebral cortex activity.

Hopefully primal woman, when she's disturbed and threatened like this, will just growl and give the look that says *don't fuck with me and my baby*. Hopefully, too, the caregiver doesn't get all huffy and officious and insistent. However, a downside of oxytocin is that, because the birthing woman is so full of these hormones and is feeling all 'friendly sweetie', she will try to comply, dragging her consciousness back through the evolutionary regression into her twenty-first-century thinking, remembering brain. It then takes us all hours to get her back down into her primal brain and instinctive rhythm.

Then there is the birthing woman's own 'stuff' to contend with. For any number of reasons her comfort zone may be narrow and restricted, so it might not take much to push her over a threshold into a discomfort zone. If she's not practised at adapting to discomfort, she may very readily spin out into a pain zone, even in early labour.

This doesn't only happen in birthing; it can be part of any demanding achievement, as Maria from performing arts troupe Strange Fruit explains:

> In terms of creative expression, because you have to work with these doubts anyway, if there's someone slightly pushing those buttons ... You don't need anyone amplifying your own self-doubts; you need them to amplify the trust.

Of course, if the birthing woman goes into her labour emotionally distressed, physically exhausted, physiologically stressed, loaded up with fear or carrying unrealistic expectations of the challenge she is facing and without any experienced support, her pain tolerance is bound to be diminished.

For some women, even though they are physically robust, psychological sabotage dynamics may also diminish pain-tolerance levels. For instance, some of us may have been emotionally patterned in our childhoods to a low pain tolerance. Maybe a way to get our dependency and nurturing needs met while growing up was to be seen to be 'suffering' and in pain.

Any unconscious relationship script with anyone in your support circle—your partner or mother particularly—where your pattern is to play the 'suffering victim' and their role is to 'rescue you', will undermine your pain-tolerance level.

So any plans for boosting your pain tolerance will need to include work to weed out any old patterns that might sabotage your intentions.

Your plans will also need to take into account the wise choices you need to make regarding your caregivers and place of birth.

Conclusion

Reframing your attitude to labour pain by understanding it as functional, physiological pain and an indication of 'things going right', rather than medical, pathological, 'things going wrong' pain, is a foundational awareness needed by all willing women.

Being motivated to work with this physiological pain and making the choices that support you and enable you to raise your pain tolerance are also essential.

Our attitudes towards pain in labour are actually highly predictive of the eventual pathway and outcome of a birth. In the next chapter we're going to look more specifically at your attitude to pain in labour—your individual 'pain type'—and what this will mean for your birth.

Personal reflection

Instinctive awareness

- To what extent does your life experience and present lifestyle support a robust instinctive awareness?
- Are you practised at recognising and acting on your instincts?
- Do you recognise when your body is calling you to move, to exert effort, to increase your heart rate in service of your stamina and fitness?
- To what extent do your instinctive needs influence the balance and rhythm of your day—what percentage of your day is directed by your body, what percentage controlled by your head or life demands?
- Do you have a particularly busy, pressured lifestyle?
- Have you begun to slow down and tune into your body?
- Has your lived experience of your instinctive body rhythms provided a solid foundation for identifying and trusting your birthing instincts?

Pain zones

- What previous experiences of raising your pain-tolerance levels will be useful to you in birthing?
- When you hit the edge of a zone—a pain-tolerance threshold—how likely are you to embrace rather than avoid, release rather than resist, accommodate rather than panic?
- Will you be able to tune into your birthing instincts through the fog of functional pain?

Birth space

- What options does your birth space offer?
- Is it enhancing or diminishing of your pain tolerance and birthing potential?

4

Approaching labour: what pain type are you?

By now you're hopefully getting clear about how the present birth culture is not user-friendly for normal physiological birthing. You're understanding more about the importance of your choices when it comes to caregivers and the place of birth. You're also now aware of the need to reframe your attitude to pain.

Now we need to go even further into the juicy topic of pain. It's time to look at your specific attitude to pain, and what this predicts for the outcome of your birth.

This is where we move out of the theory a little, and into the lived reality.

To get started, have a think about these questions: How much would you say your attitude to pain in labour, and what to do with this pain, matches up with current cultural attitudes? How much does your attitude about pain in labour match up with your family's and friends' attitudes, the attitudes of your caregivers and even the attitudes of your partner and other members of your birth team? A lot? Or not much?

Does it matter? You betcha.

Circles of influence

In chapter 3 I used the image of concentric circles when I was talking about your comfort zone. Now I want to use another set of concentric circles to help you get a sense of the influences that press in on the birthing woman when it comes to the issue of pain. The birthing woman's experience of pain in labour is influenced by her physiology and psychology and her culture—her family, friends, community and also the healthcare system and its providers.

So using the idea of these circles of influence will help you get an overall picture of the many things that have an impact on labour pain—it's not all about strong contractions.

The outer circle is the *wider cultural circle*. This 'circle of influence' is shaped by the zeitgeist, or the 'spirit of the age', and represents cultural biases, including all those 'labour-bypass era' inclinations.

Inside this circle is the *wider circle of family and friends*—their attitudes, stories and suggestions.

Inside this circle is the *circle of birth-place culture*, with its practices and procedures regarding pain.

Finally, there is the *circle of known support*. This innermost circle of influence refers to who you have with you during the birth and their 'take' on pain.

At the centre of all these circles, with all the attitudes, stories, practices and influences about pain that they represent, sits the birthing woman with her lived experience of her own comfort, discomfort and pain zones.

Circles of Influence (Fig 4.1)

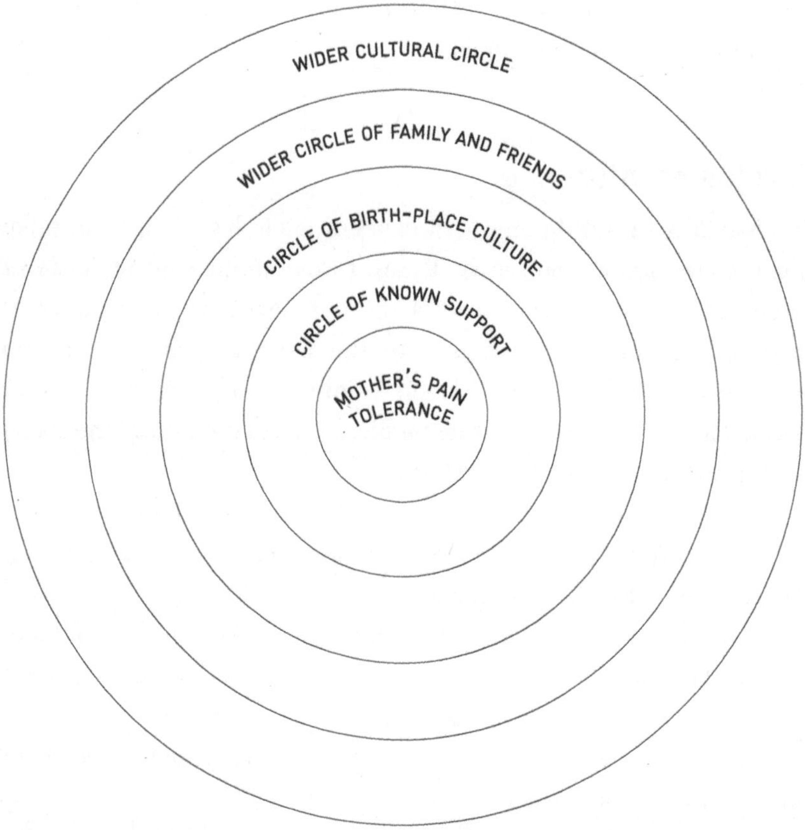

Wider cultural circle

I spoke a lot about the attitudes contained in this circle in the last chapter, so I'm pretty sure you know what you are up against here. If not, just start chatting to anybody in the supermarket checkout line, or pregnancy clinic, or doctor's waiting room—or anywhere really. Talk to them about your plans for normal physiological birth, how you're just going to breathe your way through labour, and I'm sure you'll get the cultural message loud and clear!

Whether you like it or not, these negative undermining messages about pain also take up space in your own head and psyche.[48] In the main, willing women need to protect themselves from this way of thinking and supplant that undermining mindset with a new one, by reframing their attitude to pain as suggested in chapter 3.

But when push comes to shove and you hit moments of vulnerability during labour, what happens? Imagine a moment of vulnerability when you hit an overwhelming pain barrier and you want out. You want the drugs and you want them now! The floodgates in your psyche open and all the acculturated ways of thinking about pain come flooding in. Then what?

If you follow these embedded cultural messages then pain-relief thinking takes over. Will you be at the mercy of this thinking, or will you have a buffer zone to protect you from it?

Wider circle of family and friends

When the birthing woman hits a pain barrier she will be far more likely to overcome it if she has a buffer zone provided by her own *wider circle of family and friends* protecting her from those negative cultural influences lurking in her psyche.

The *wider circle of family and friends* is made up of 'her people'. Not the ones she will have with her at the birth, but all her other close family and friends who are there with her in the form of stories, comments, suggestions and attitudes.

Do they moderate the cultural message and provide a buffer zone of protection from the acculturated inner voice? Or do they amp up the cultural message in her head and reaffirm that she was stupid to ever think she could do it without an epidural?

If this *wider circle of family and friends* doesn't provide a buffer zone for the struggling birthing woman to lean into, it will instead act as an amplifier and multiplier of the acculturated 'pain-relief' mindset. *Now* what's going to happen?

This is where the philosophy and practice within your chosen birth place comes to the fore.

Circle of birth-place culture

In our present birth systems, apart from in small pockets, the *circle of birth-place culture* will predominately be made up of people who are strangers to the birthing woman—all the midwives and obstetric teams that make up the institutional 'stranger caregivers' who attend the mother. Relationships with members of this 'circle of influence' are forged due to institutional circumstance and who is on the roster at the time. As well as people, this circle also includes the philosophies, routines, practices, power relationships and workplace regulations of the place of birth, which influence not only who will be working with you but also how they work.

The concept of 'birth territory' (also referred to in chapter 3), is described by midwifery researchers, educators and editors, Kathleen Fahy, Maralyn Foureur and Carolyn Hastie, as dealing 'with the physical, the social and the metaphysical space and the issue of power concerning who is in control of the space'.[49] This concept overlaps with my idea of this *circle of birth-place culture*, although here I'm particularly focusing on how this influences the birthing woman's approach to pain.

I'm sure you can see how important your choices are. Have you ensured that your caregivers are aware of your intentions for normal physiological birth? Are you sure they know how to back up your intentions by offering that buffer zone—the expertise to lean into during any pain panic moments?

Or are your caregivers more used to fulfilling the promise offered by a pain-relief, pain-free mindset and so most likely to offer the drugs that can save you from the painful effort? If that's the case then it's going to fall to your *circle of known support* to help. What sort of buffer between you and the drugs can they provide?

Circle of known support

This *circle of known support* is made up of the people the birthing woman is *choosing* to have with her—people who are known to her, usually her partner and perhaps some other family members or friends.

The circle may also include particular caregivers she is engaging for the birth, such as a 'known' or 'named' midwife, a birth attendant/doula, or a private obstetrician. (Just a point here: although I'm including private obstetricians in this known group, they do not really fulfil a pain-support function. Obstetricians do not take an active role in the hour-by-hour, contraction-by-contraction, breath-by-breath work of birth support.)

The birthing woman will have many motivations for choosing the known birth companions who make up her circle of known support. Her motivations might be shaped by social or cultural expectations or external pressures. Or her choices may have been arrived at after much savvy deliberation.

I separate this *circle of known support* into two distinct kinds: the *naïve support circle* and the *facilitating holding circle*.

The *naïve support circle* is, either by design or by default, set up in such a way that the birthing woman will be encouraged to access pain-relief options in order to be 'saved' when a pain crisis hits. In the moments of a crisis of confidence, when she herself wants all the drugs she can get, perhaps her partner or her mother will actually be the mouthpiece for the familiar cultural messages—'Oh, you poor thing you shouldn't have to suffer like this', 'See? It's not possible', or 'I told you so'. This can occur whether the birthing woman was initially a 'willing woman' or not.

The *naïve support circle* is distinct from the *facilitating holding circle*. The *facilitating holding circle* is specifically designed by a *savvy* willing woman to support her through pain and distress barriers, in order to back her intentions for normal physiological birth.

If our cultural messages about pain in labour have been multiplied by her *wider support circle of family and friends* and then reinforced by the *birth place culture*, then these messages are all going to come rushing in, swamping even the willing woman's original intentions and confirming her present distressed self-talk. 'I can't do it!' she wails.

Now it's going to fall to this *circle of known support* to hold the line if the willing woman's original intentions are to be honoured. Is there any buffer zone? Any protective force field within this inner circle, protecting her from both her own self-doubts and the multiplied, magnified messages of the culture? Is there anything to protect her from the cultural messages that say, 'No, you can't do it and anyway you don't have to'?

Unfortunately, these various circles of influence generally set up a negative pressure. The whole system is applying pressure inwards on the birthing woman, who is feeling shaky and vulnerable about pain anyway. The messages that usually come at her say, 'You can be comfortable. No, you can't do it. No, you're silly for even thinking that you can. No, you don't need to do it. No, don't be a martyr. Yes, you should be comfortable.'

It's *so* important who you choose for your support team. Have you got on board a *naïve support circle* who will, in the testing moments, become the negative enablers of the pain-relief mindset? Or do you have people with the stamina, attitudes and expertise to act as a *facilitating holding circle*?

Buffer or sabotage?

For our birthing woman, whether she's a willing woman at the onset of labour or not, when she's hitting a pain panic—a moment of vulnerability—how many circles can she lean into to buffer the sabotaging cultural mindset? Will any of the circles hold for her and provide a positive, energetic buffer? Will any amplify a positive message and back up her intentions for normal physiological birthing?

Or will all those negative attitudes come rushing in, multiplying and building as they crash through circle after circle, like a snowball rolling downhill gathering speed—to eventually crash through the willing woman's now flimsy-seeming intentions?

Hopefully a willing woman is blessed with a *wider circle of family and friends* who can provide at least the initial much-needed buffer from the negative cultural messages. Then the savvy willing woman can, by her choices, increase the buffer zone and back herself by ensuring she has a birth-place culture and a *facilitating holding circle* that match her intentions.

Unfortunately though, most women do not have the kinds of circles of influence that would support them for normal physiological birth. In fact, very few are even aware that they will need them. Some willing women may believe that their own attitudes to pain, their own intentions for normal physiological childbirth will be enough to see them through the work of labour. But in my experience, this is not enough.

In the absence of any buffer zone provided by her support team, place of birth or family and friends, can the willing woman hold herself? She may expect her personal attitude to pain in labour to give her a buffer zone in her own head, but without carefully chosen circles of support and with all that negative cultural pressure pressing in on her, it will be tough to stay with her own intentions.

This isn't to say that a woman's own attitude to pain in labour isn't important though. The birthing woman's attitude to pain provides the portal through which all the positive or negative messages from the circles of influence will flow. Her attitude dictates how strongly these messages will take up residence in her psyche.

Pain dynamics

As well as being aware of the circles of influence, it is also important that a willing woman understands something of the pain dynamics of birth. What do I mean by pain dynamics? In writing this phrase I am referring to the interplay between the birthing woman, her caregivers and her support team when she hits a pain barrier—the reactions of those around her when she reaches a point where she feels she can't go on.

When a birthing woman reaches such a barrier or threshold, this can set off a 'crisis of confidence', which leads her to want out of the whole deal. I've mentioned this idea of a crisis of confidence earlier and will be expanding on it at length in chapter 5. Here I just need to say again that this 'crisis of confidence' experience has a great impact on how the birth will eventually turn out. To be clear, what I'm calling a crisis of confidence is not to be confused with 'transition' (8–10 cm) at the end of first stage. But, like transition, crises of confidence are predictable.

When a woman reaches a crisis of confidence, those around her can react in a number of ways. In this situation, a willing woman needs support from these people to continue working through her distress. What will her support team do? Are they able to tap her strength and support her through? Or are they going to be triggered into pity and want to save her?

The 'pain is power' metaphor I mentioned in chapter 3 is also important to bear in mind here. In this situation, whoever manages the pain will gain power over the circumstances of the birth.

When these pain dynamics get going and the birthing woman is in this crisis of confidence, her attitude to pain in labour will be laid bare and the feelings, attitudes, skills and intentions of the people around her will also be revealed.

Your pain type

In the last chapter I spoke about the need for a major reframing of your thinking about pain in labour. Hopefully, you have started this process of adjusting your view of pain in labour and can view it as a healthy, functional process to be embraced and worked with. If you have—great! But I'm sorry to have to tell you that your work's not over yet. Because guess what? Pain in labour is *still pain*.

You can have the healthiest possible attitude to pain in labour, but it's still going to hurt! So, this is where I'll ask you to have a think about your own personal 'pain type'. How do you usually deal with functional pain? Do you usually avoid it altogether? Can you manage a little but like to stay within a limited comfort zone? Or do you embrace it wholeheartedly?

It's worth working out just what your pain type is, because in my experience these 'types' help to explain what happens when pain dynamics get going in labour.

The following types apply specifically to a birthing woman's attitude towards pain. However, in many cases her pain attitude may overlap with her overall attitude about birth. For instance, because they are aware of the high intervention rates, many women take a 'wait and see' approach. Their attitude is: 'let's not get fixated on the way the birth goes. Let's just see what happens.' For a willing woman in a birth culture that fully supported normal physiological birth this might make sense. The woman would wait and see if any true medical need for intervention arose. But in the present labour-bypass era this passive approach to the birth is akin to signing up for the inevitable cascade of interventions.

No, the willing woman needs to be *proactive*. She needs to be focused on the wise choices—of birth place, caregivers and experienced support—that will back her intentions for normal physiological birth. Then, and only then, when all that is in place, will an overall 'wait and see' attitude be an expression of an appropriate surrender to the unfolding circumstances of the birth mystery.

Okay, so what's your attitude?

Over the years of my involvement in birth work I've become aware of five 'attitude groups' when it comes to pain in labour. These can help to predict what will happen when pain dynamics get going. Spread across a continuum they are a 'pain-avoiding' group, a 'status quo' group, a 'wait and see' group, an 'aspirational but naïve' group, and, finally, a 'pain embracing' group.

Pain-avoiding attitude

These women take a proactive position—proactive to *avoid* all pain in labour. Women who have this attitude hit a 'crisis of confidence' long before the labour. They've taken the cultural message about pain in labour and run with it. They're highly motivated to avoid all pain and have made the particular choices that back their intentions for a managed, pain-free labour. They don't want to leave it to chance, they want that 'epidural at the first contraction', or possibly even an elective caesarean.

They see no value in the pain of labour or working with it and instead feel that 'in this day and age women shouldn't have to suffer the barbaric pain of labour'. For these women, the epidural has it covered and they're damn well going to get one.

This position is a combination of other attitudes—that modern medicine should be able to save us from the ordeal of pain, and that, anyway, it's our right to choose. This can also combine with feminist ideals about freeing women from the burdens of our reproductive maternal bodies.

This *pain-avoiding woman* is highly motivated to avoid all pain in labour; she's fearful of the pain, sees no value in it and wants it fully controlled. She ensures she is definitely surrounded by 'pain relief' attitudes and practices—she is not leaving it to chance. She makes particular choices regarding place of birth and caregivers and definitely does not want to 'lose control'. She wants a 'civilised' birth and so plans to avoid any of that messy crisis vulnerability stuff.

She doesn't want to deal with the pain, she doesn't see that she should have to, it's not on her agenda. This attitude is entirely backed by the current cultural mindset and birth culture practices. This attitude is incompatible with a willing woman's intentions.

'Status quo' attitude

These women take an acquiescent position—acquiescent to the dominant cultural and medical messages. They are acquiescent to anyone they perceive is an expert—their caregivers, neighbours, friends … just about anybody, really. With this trusting acquiescence, the issue of pain-management choices is shaped by whatever advice is offered.

The *status-quo woman* is particularly acquiescent to the dominant 'pain-relief' paradigm and practices. In fact, she's usually unaware that there is any other choice. She is unable to normalise any 'crisis' vulnerabilities and having taken in the cultured message is too fearful of the pain to see any value in working with it as a capacity-building process.

Her attitude runs something like this: 'Well, I don't know what to do, so I'm just going to listen to the experts', or 'Everyone says epidurals are the way to go, so I guess that's what I'll need'.

When I originally began to refine my understanding of these dynamics, *status quo women* were not as likely to be 'nudged' towards the epidural. Back then, *pain-avoiding women* were definitely pushing the boundaries of the accepted norms about pain-management in labour—they were the early adopters of epidurals. Now, with the shift of epidural use from 'medical need' to an option of 'social choice', this status quo group, encouraged by the experts surrounding them, is merging with the pain-avoiding group in terms of the kind of birth outcome they can expect.

'Wait and see' attitude

These women have a wavering position. They have some yearning for normal physiological birth and, although they have a sense that there may be a way to work with the physiological pain, they also sense the enormity of the challenge—so they hedge their bets.

The *'wait and see' woman*'s attitude is underpinned, like many other women's, by a belief that pain thresholds are set at a particular point. A woman in this group doesn't realise that her pain tolerance can be influenced up or down by many factors, including the type of support she receives.

Her attitude runs something like this: 'You know, women have been birthing forever and they even go back for more, so it can't be that bad—there's got to be something going for it. And I've heard there are some hormones that can help. On the other hand, I've heard stories ... maybe it's not so easy as all that. I think I have a pretty good pain threshold, I hardly ever use pain killers, except maybe something for a headache or period pain, and I push myself a bit at the gym or hiking, so probably I'll be okay. But I just don't know how painful it will be and whether my pain threshold will match it. I have doubts and fears in the back of my mind so I'm thinking I'll just wait and see how it goes. I'm not going to be a martyr about it, I'll just wait till I'm in it, then I'll make some decisions about what I'll do.'

So here's a set-up for pain relief, because when the going gets tough the default nature of pain-relief management practices will mean this *'wait and see' woman* is offered and accepts the drugs.

The *'wait and see' woman* is unsure whether her pain threshold will match the demands of labour; she is prepared to work with pain till her pain threshold is reached. If that's enough to get her through, well then, okay; if not, she will make decisions about pain management in the moment. This woman is unable to normalise 'crisis' vulnerabilities and doesn't understand that she can use support to raise her pain tolerance, so she doesn't pay attention to appropriate support needs. She doesn't have awareness of the implications of different pain-management ideas and has only a marginal feeling that working with pain has value as a capacity-building process.

Aspirational but naïve attitude

These women take a proactive stance based on their personal power. They are actively preparing for the birth; they've done their homework. They are willing women, they expect a normal physiological birth and they may even have made some wise choices. But they are naïve about the realities of 'the system', the realities of the pressure from the circles of influence and about the potency of pain and pain dynamics in labour.

The *aspirational but naïve woman* is motivated for normal physiological birth but is unrealistic regarding the challenge; she is self-reliant, into self-control and may buy into the 'pain-free' story offered by some birth preparation techniques. She is in denial about 'crisis' vulnerabilities because she believes they are never going to happen to her. Because of this, she doesn't pay attention to the need for experienced support. Finally, she sees overcoming the pain as a mark of her sense of self and an expression of her personal power.

The *aspirational but naïve woman*'s attitude goes: 'Well, women are the stronger sex and birthing women are powerful goddesses. They give birth in caves, under trees, up trees in the middle of floods, in cars, here and there, everywhere. And anyway, look at me! I'm a fantastic example of a woman, I'm fit and healthy, a can-do woman. Besides, I've done my reading, I'm exercising, practising my breathing, my stretching, my relaxation, my hypno therapy techniques, my birth skills; I do pregnancy yoga, I'm walking and swimming, taking raspberry leaf tea. If any woman can do it I can! Bring it on!'

These are willing women, they aspire to the experience of normal physiological birth, but they are naïve about three things—the impact of the circles of influence flooding them at crucial moments; the reality of the high intervention rates brought on by labour-bypass era practices (in their eyes those interventions only happen to 'the women who haven't got their act together'), and, lastly, they are naïve about the 'crisis of confidence' moments that activate pain dynamics.

The *aspirational but naïve woman* believes that just by saying 'I've made it clear in my birth plan that I don't want any drugs and definitely no epidural', she has done enough to protect herself from the seduction of the epidural and its consequences, even if she is in a private hospital with an epidural rate running at 80% and a caesarean rate over 50%.

'It's never going to happen to me, I'm never going to be pleading for an epidural, it only happens to those other wimpy women', thinks the *aspirational but naïve woman*. She sees the birth experience as being all within her own power and control, so she doesn't pay enough attention to her birth choices or support team. In fact, she's often choosing entirely inappropriate people to support her—perhaps her sister who has had two epidurals (because she wants to show her how a 'real' woman should do it). Or she relies entirely on her inexperienced partner because she wants just an intimate experience. This sounds romantic doesn't it? I can certainly understand the yearning for an intimate experience with the father of your baby. But trust me when I tell you that this is an incredibly naïve approach to your support needs in labour and one that will not serve the willing woman well in her efforts to avoid interventions.

At the point of a crisis of confidence, when her self-belief starts to crumble, this woman's aspirations can disintegrate quickly because she and her equally naïve support team are not able to normalise any crisis of confidence. When one hits and she's pleading for pain relief, they all feel there must be something going terribly wrong.

The *aspirational but naïve woman* has not fully grasped that the issue of pain in labour is a social, cultural and structural issue, not just an issue of her own personal power and control.

Looking back at myself before my first daughter's birth I can identify with this group. In fact, I would take it a step further and say that, not only was I an *aspirational but naïve woman*, I was an *arrogant* one!

Pain-embracing attitude

These women take a proactive stance based on their personal power, enhanced by experienced support. These women are willing women—*savvy* willing women.

They are highly motivated toward normal physiological birth and they know that pain is its territory. They understand that 'pain is power' not only physically but also in the power play that surrounds a birthing woman. They accept the challenge of embracing the intensity, conscious of the enormity of the task.

They understand the lessons from the 'circles of influence' and have made wise choices about their birth-place culture and their facilitating holding circle. They have reflected on the psychological and physiological impact of the pain dynamics and how these might manifest in their particular story and have prepared themselves and strengthened their birth circles accordingly.

They have put as much (psychic and physical) distance as they can between themselves and the seduction of the epidural and have designed safety plans in the event that this space seems to close in during a crisis of confidence. They know they will hit crises of confidence, so they are specifically planning and preparing beforehand for crisis moments. They have done 'the work', physically and psychologically, and feel ready for the challenge, while also keeping an awareness of the need for flexibility in the face of the unknown.

The *pain-embracing woman* understands the negative impact of the dominant birth culture on her birthing potential, the way it can undermine her resolve in crisis of confidence moments. She understands the need for midwifery care and experienced support to hold her to her intentions in these moments. Generally, this group makes choices outside the social norm—maybe birth centres, 'know your midwife' or 'named' midwife schemes or homebirths. Or, if they make the more usual public labour ward or private hospital choices, they strengthen their *facilitating holding circle* with experienced support, in order to protect their intentions about working with pain.

The *pain-embracing woman*, being highly motivated for normal physiological birth and consequently realistic regarding the need to work with pain in labour, make specific choices to ensure that she is definitely surrounded by 'working with pain' practices, attitudes and expertise. She makes particular choices regarding place of birth and caregivers; is expecting 'crisis' moments and therefore understands she will need experienced support. The *pain-embracing woman* also develops her own skills and resources, and values 'working with pain' as a capacity-building process.

Like their pain-avoiding sisters at the opposite end of the spectrum, these women are not leaving it to chance. They are making the choices to ensure they have the expertise they need with them.

The *pain-embracing woman* and the *aspirational but naïve woman* share some similarities. They may undertake some of the same preparation. The main difference is their awareness of crisis of confidence dynamics and of the importance of having the right people in their circle of known support. This is what makes the crucial difference.

As part of their preparation for the birth, both the *aspirational but naïve* and the *pain-embracing woman* will have practised breathing and relaxation techniques. However, they will be coming at these techniques from different perspectives. For the *aspirational but naïve woman* the motivation for these practices is a desire to avoid pain. She wants the techniques to deliver a pain-free experience. As I've already explained, this leaves her very vulnerable to an epidural if the practised techniques do not deliver on the pain-free promise. The *pain-embracing woman* on the other hand understands that any breathing and relaxation techniques are resources for boosting her pain tolerance and for working into the expected functional pain of normal physiological birth. She is under no illusions about the fact that she will have to work *with* it.

Where do you sit?

These five groups of women are not equal in numbers.

Since I first began using this model to explain the pathways that are set in play around pain, the social norm has shifted away from the 'embrace pain' end of the continuum. At that time (in the late eighties, early nineties) there were only a small number of 'radical' pain-avoiding women hunting down the epidurals. Now the numbers are weighted in the opposite direction, with the 'radical' women being the 'pain embracing' group.

Okay, do you recognise yourself? Where do you place yourself on this continuum of attitudes?

Pain attitudes (Fig 4.2)

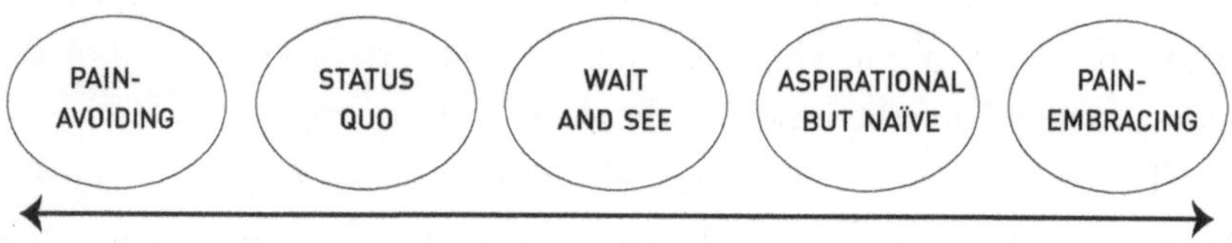

Keep this in mind, because after I've explained some other influences on the birth relating to pain I'm going to predict the pathway of your birth based on your pain type.

Also remember that, at the point of a crisis of confidence, birthing women want all those drugs. So it will depend on who is around her—what buffer is provided, or not—as to whether she accesses them. For this reason, a birthing woman's partner and other support people will also need to reflect on *their* attitudes to pain.

Are they aligned with you?

Your midwife's attitude to pain

As already mentioned, the midwife plays a pivotal role in the way these pain dynamics will unfold.

Research by midwifery academic Nicky Leap into midwives' attitudes to labour pain illustrates the reason the midwife counts so much when it comes to pain in labour. Her research identified two distinct midwifery attitudes to pain in labour—a 'pain relief' paradigm and a 'working with pain' paradigm.[50 51 52]

The midwife may be an independent midwife specifically chosen by you, or she may be the midwife who has made a relationship with you through the pregnancy, after being assigned to you through a 'know your midwife' or 'named midwife' program. Or she may be the 'stranger' midwife who happens to be on shift at the time.

Midwives are generally caring and nurturing, with excellent people skills. So, in describing more fully Nicky Leap's research into midwives' attitudes to pain in labour, I am not making comment on their caring qualities or commitment to women and babies. This research is about fundamental differences in understanding pain in childbirth—differences that have major consequences for a woman's birthing potential.

Willing women need to understand the implications of this research in order to back their intentions for normal physiological birth.

Pain-relief paradigm

This way of thinking is informed by medical and nursing models that underpin obstetric thinking and dominate most hospital birth settings. This is a paradigm based on pain-relief management developed for *pathological* pain in nursing, medicine, emergency and surgery situations—you know, the 'assess your pain between one and ten' routine. The bottom line for this way of thinking is that pain should be controlled so that you can remain 'comfortable'.

The experts at managing pathological pain are anaesthetists, medical caregivers, chemists, nurses and those midwives who are influenced by this pain-relief paradigm. They know about the drugs and the epidurals—the 'when', 'how' and 'how much'.

The approach of those working within this paradigm when it comes to birthing leads labouring women to the 'pain relief menu'—designed to keep you comfortable so you don't 'suffer' unnecessarily. The menu consists of pharmacological methods of pain relief (entenox, pethidine or equivalent opiate and epidural anaesthesia), with many birthing women going through the entire menu from entrée to main course to dessert.

The views of those working in this model are based on the belief that the importance of women being comfortable and pain free, outweighs any of the disadvantages, risks and unintended consequences of pharmacological pain relief. (Besides, caregivers are used to picking up the pieces medically if it all goes pear-shaped.) Amberley says:

> I had an epidural, and ten minutes later the baby's heart rate dropped and eight doctors walked in and dragged our baby out.

Sari tells a similar story:

> After the epidural the heartbeat became irregular and the obstetrician was called back and (the birth) ended up in an emergency c-section.

Hospitals, and therefore most birth settings, are dominated by this pain-relief thinking. In these situations, any distress on hitting points of vulnerability, pain barriers or crises of confidence, instead of being normalised and supported, will become entry points for the pain-relief options. These options are supposedly offered in the spirit of 'informed choice', but in reality, in these care settings, with an absence of any other meaningful support for boosting pain tolerance, they actually work as 'nudge' choices and are almost impossible to opt out of, as the following illustrates. Anna's sister-in-law describes Anna's typical 'cascade birth':

> Anna had no hope, they just bombarded her. I was staggered at the number of times she was offered pain relief before she'd even got into strong labour. So eventually she gave in.

Erin, who we first met in chapter 2, also unfortunately met a 'pain relief' midwife at a point of distress:

> The syntocin-fired contractions had no natural ebb and flow and the midwife suggested an epidural. I somehow agreed to it—a place I did not want to go. When I look back now I realise it was the only thing offered to me at that time. I am disappointed that at that point of distress I was not encouraged to try something else—as I had wanted—and couldn't advocate for my needs better.[53]

This pain-relief paradigm is a perfect philosophical match for the *pain-avoiding woman*, who is definitely seeking out this midwife and the pain-relief birth culture. Also, because this paradigm is the dominant one, '*status quo*', '*wait and see*' and '*aspirational but naïve*' *women* will generally, by default, find themselves with these midwives. The *pain-embracing woman*, in contrast, is protecting herself from this way of thinking and doesn't want to leave it to chance that a midwife with this attitude might attend her in labour.

'Working with pain' paradigm

In contrast to the medically influenced pain-relief practices, a 'working with pain' philosophy comes out of 'keeping birth normal' midwifery models.

This philosophy is underpinned by two core beliefs. Firstly, that normal physiological birth takes normal physiological pain and that, with the right support, women can work with that pain. Secondly, that functional pain plays an important role in the physiology of normal labour because, as mentioned previously, functional pain is a stimulator of endorphins, which are part of the hormonal cascade that promotes normal physiological birth, as well as the complex mix of hormones that enhances 'bonding behaviours' towards babies.

'Working with pain' in labour, just like working with functional pain in other endeavours, requires practical skills and summons intense human support. Experts in these forms of support are personal trainers, coaches, yoga teachers, massage therapists, sports psychologists, team mates and so on—and, when it comes to birthing, the experts are midwives who are influenced by this paradigm and experienced birth attendants or doulas. (Or maybe they are your mother, sister or best friend who has climbed this mountain before you.)

When birthing women are well supported by midwives who embody this 'working with pain' philosophy, they will be encouraged *through* pain barriers, supported through any vulnerability or crisis moments and guided into a deeper rhythm of engagement with their body, facilitating the emergence of their birthing power.

Now there is a need, obviously, to be able to discern the difference between normal (physiological) and abnormal (pathological) pain states in labour. However, indications of pathology in labour are not very often signalled by pain, rather they are signalled by physiological markers (pulse rate, blood pressure, blood loss, baby's heart rate and others). As a general rule, you can trust the pain in all its intensity and give expression to the pain, because your physiological sounds, your singing—what I call the 'song of the cervix' sounds—give clues to your labour's progress.

The *pain-embracing woman* is definitely choosing midwives with these 'working with pain' skills. They make a perfect philosophical match. Also, any of the *'status quo'*, *'wait and see'*, or *'aspirational but naïve' women* who are willing women will have got lucky if they happen to come across this 'working with pain' midwife, because she will be able to support and guide them through any crisis.

Pain-avoiding women, on the other hand, don't want to go anywhere near this 'working with pain' midwife. They don't want to leave it to chance that they might run up against her. They are making sure that they access a 'pain-relief' midwife; they don't want a midwife trying to talk them through any crisis of confidence thank you, they just want the epidural.

The impact of the midwife

Whoever the midwife is and whatever your contact with her, there are many aspects to her care that are going to have an impact on your birthing capacity.

In particular, you will want to work out if she is a midwife who fits the mould as a 'new' midwife, a facilitating midwife for normal physiological birth. Or if she is a midwife more attuned to nursing techno-medical-based practices. Do you know? How will you work it out?

Does it matter? You betcha.

Let's imagine a typical situation. A birthing woman hits a crisis of confidence. She is distressed and feeling she can't go on. 'I can't do it', she wails. 'Help me, help me, get me something.' She is weeping and imploring her support team to give her the drugs or an epidural. Regardless of her intentions before the birth, now she wants out.

If she is birthing in a birth setting dominated by a pain-relief practice, or is attended in these crucial crisis moments by a midwife with a pain-relief attitude and practice, her emotional distress and crisis will be interpreted by her midwife as 'unnecessary suffering'. Then, being a caring midwife within this pain-relief paradigm, this midwife will feel that her best duty of care for the birthing woman at these crisis moments is to 'save' her from that suffering. The way she can do that is by offering the birthing woman the 'pain-relief menu'. Then the birthing woman, in her distress, and in the absence of any other buffer, will gratefully accept the smorgasbord on offer.

On the other hand, if the woman is birthing in a care setting based on the 'working with pain' model, or if, in any crisis moments, she is attended by a midwife whose practice is informed by a 'working with pain' philosophy, the midwife will respond differently.

Far from seeing you as 'suffering', she will see 'potency'. In fact, she has been waiting to see these moments of vulnerability come forward because she knows that they are signs of progress. These crisis moments of vulnerability are a sign that the hormones and contractions are intensifying. So the midwife is celebrating this intensity jump-up. She is settling you, supporting, encouraging and boosting your pain tolerance, and then guiding you into a deeper engagement with your labour.

It's not rocket science; it's very easy to see the different probable outcomes in these scenarios. Same woman, same pain vulnerabilities but different possibilities based on the midwifery support she recieves.

Research reported in *Pain in Childbearing and its Control*[54] supports this understanding. This research came from Denmark. The researchers were able to follow two groups of women and compare their behaviours in labour and their birth outcomes. All the women in the study were matched and had intentions to birth in an Alternative Birth Centre (ABC), which meant they were all initially willing women who had intentions for normal physiological birth. However, because of the popularity and size of the birth centre some women were refused admission and had to birth in the 'obstetrical ward'. Keep in mind that these women were not 'transferred' out of the birth centre because of any medical need, they just couldn't all fit in.

So, it was a handy group to study to see the impact of birth-place culture and pain-management practice on the birthing woman's initial resolve. Would her pain tolerance be raised or lowered? Would she be supported through the pain or saved from it? Well, the women unable to use the birth centre ended up matching the 'obstetric ward' women (those who had chosen the obstetric ward in the first place) in both their behaviour in labour and the interventions they received—they conformed to the obstetric ward practices. 'Thus the culture of the obstetrical ward staff and the environment in which they practised was demonstrated to have overcome the aspirations and education of the ABC-refused women,' the research stated.

Willing women need to be savvy about this. If they are birthing with stranger midwives, willing women need to make sure that their own *facilitating holding circle* has expertise to protect them from pain-relief thinking and practices—as well as the expertise to come close and support them through any crises of confidence.

Giving your midwife 'the green light'

One way a willing woman can draw out a 'working with pain' midwife is by giving a clear green light on her birth plan. Or even by writing specifically to the head of midwifery at her hospital, as in the following letter:

> Dear Head of Midwifery
>
> You recommended that I write a little of my past experiences as well as my hopes for this impending birth, as it will be my third baby but only my first delivery at your hospital. My previous labours were problematic in areas relating to the support provided in the labour ward, and I am anxious to avoid these issues recurring if at all possible.
>
> My first labour took forty hours. At that time I did not know about posterior presentations, spurious labour or that I could expect more from my midwife when she said she'd be at the desk if I needed her! Labour ended with an epidural and ventouse extraction, two doses of pethidine and a very sleepy baby who failed to attach for breastfeeding for several days.
>
> My second labour took twenty hours with only two and a half in the labour ward before delivery. On this occasion there was no time for pain relief—it was fast and furious. An unsympathetic midwife jabbed at me with her long finger nails and complained to my obstetrician that if I'd just relax I could have had the baby fifteen minutes earlier!
>
> Apart from my obvious desire to have a healthy child, my overwhelming want, this time, is to come out of this labour with some sense of achievement, fulfilment or peace rather than trauma and shock.
>
> In my previous two labours I have felt at war with my body, that I was a victim of desperate pain that I could do little to overcome and had no one to help change the situation. With regard to the last comment, I feel the absence of midwife

support was critical to my experience and overall quite lacking. While I have an extremely supportive husband who supported me endlessly, he is a man who had no previous experience of labour and could do little in the way of providing information and encouragement as I progressed or failed to progress through my labours.

The World Health Organization quotes research, which shows that continuous empathetic and physical support during labour results in shorter labour, less medication, fewer epidurals and operative deliveries and higher Apgar scores. It is the experience that midwives have that I would hope to draw on for this labour, so that I can feel my midwife is supporting the journey alongside of me, providing me with simple but constant encouragement and information. To remind me that my body is doing exactly what it should, that I am making progress, that I could try different positions to help manage the pain better. I need to be kept present and participating rather than feeling completely lost, paralysed with fear and wanting to be as far away from the labour as possible. I hope that my midwife and my husband can help me to find the strength from deep within me to birth my baby safely and without medical intervention.

We accept that labour is painful but want to work with that pain.

We recognise that movement and positioning are key in managing labour and ask for as much suggestion and support in choosing and carrying out positions for an active birth. When I chose to deliver on all fours for my second baby, it was made quite clear that this was not desirable from the midwives' point of view. This attitude, we feel, is really quite inappropriate.

While my husband intends to be a very active support person, we recognise that the midwives' support is invaluable and expect that as far as possible they will be available throughout labour to provide this to us both.

In view of our past experiences we have also decided to bring with us an extra support person, whom we expect will be welcomed and respected for her own expertise.

Kind regards
Maude

Willing women need to identify themselves to their entire birth team, including the stranger midwife, by giving a green light on their birth plan in order to draw out a 'working with pain' midwife. These midwives are hungry to work with willing women; they would love to work with a woman who wants to be active and engage with her body.

On their part, to make sure of the philosophical match, these midwives need to be able to identify if you are a willing women as well. After all, when birthing women are in a crisis of confidence they pretty well all look and sound the same. So the midwife needs to know beforehand what your intentions are. Are you a willing woman who wants to be supported through a crisis of confidence? Or are you a pain-avoiding woman who just wants the epidural, no question about it?

As Associate Professor of Midwifery from the University of Western Sydney Hannah Dahlen says, 'Perhaps then, the right woman will give birth in the right place at the right time and with the right health care provider and have outcomes that are both safe and satisfying'.[55]

It would certainly be wonderful if we could avoid the frustrations and mixed agendas present in the following scenarios, described by a midwife in a letter to me:

> I appreciate that you are so realistic when you present … people really do need to know what goes on when birth takes place in hospitals. It is a privilege, but very difficult to work with women other than the 'embracing pain' fully determined woman. There is so much pressure when working within the system to conform to rules and protocols and time schedules. Some of us are out there trying to be 'with woman' and we get incident reports written about us for 'talking the woman out of an epidural'.

I will take on board the suggestion of speaking with the pregnant woman and her partner prior to labour, if I know the woman, or as early in the labour as I can, if the woman is unknown to me.

Regards Joan

The perils of leaving it to chance

Another point: midwifery shifts in hospital are generally eight to ten hours long, (7 am to 3 pm, 2 pm to 10 pm, 9.30 pm to 7.30 am), which is generally not long enough to cover a birth, particularly a first birth. (If we were really setting up the birth system to support normal physiological birth we would structure this differently, which does happen in some situations.)

In most care settings, for a first birth, you need to assume that you will be working with more than one midwife. Most likely, you will have a midwife for the end of her shift then another for a full shift then maybe even go into the start of another shift. This means you may be working with a minimum of two midwives and up to eight or nine different midwives, if you take into account lunch and dinner breaks and the other midwives who cover these break times.

Holding the precarious edge with a birthing woman in the throes of a crisis of confidence requires intense consistent support. Because of the dominance of pain-relief practice, I can assure you that in no hospital setting, apart from in very small pockets, are you definitely going to get lucky and be assigned two, three, four or more 'working with pain' midwives in a row.

In fact, these 'working with pain' midwives tell me that they dare not go on their lunch break, because they know that when they get back, the covering midwife, who is likely to be a 'pain-relief' midwife, will have the epidural organised.

So, it's not only about choosing between different birth-place cultures, it's also important to understand the differences within a particular birth place. Sally's story highlights these differences and their possible consequences:

> Gennie [midwife], I used your optimism that it was possible for me to handle the pain of the contractions. I appreciated your calm support and presence through the contractions, your acceptance of the way I handled my contractions and your support for me doing whatever I was doing at the time. This was in stark contrast to the midwifery support I had after your shift finished, which meant that within an hour of you leaving I was having an epidural. Very quickly after being given the epidural, the baby's heart rate went down and I was rushed to theatre for a caesarean.

If you are birthing in these settings and you are a savvy willing woman you can see how important it is to not leave it to chance, but instead to make sure you have this 'working with pain' expertise in your *facilitating holding circle*. In this labour-bypass era you cannot leave it to chance that the birthing goddesses will shine on you and organise a consistent run of stranger 'working with pain' midwives.

I'm building up a picture of all the players involved in these pain dynamics. We have the birthing woman with her attitude to pain; we have her birth team with their attitudes; we have the midwife, either a 'pain-relief' or 'working with pain' midwife and we have the birth place culture. Then they are all swept up in the heaving seas and storms of a crisis of confidence. Let's see what washes up.

Predicted birth outcomes

Choices have consequences. Based on the birthing woman's attitude to pain and the structural issues pressing in on her, I imagine that by now you, too, can predict what's going to happen to the labour when a crisis of confidence gets going.

These predictions are based on the present birth culture, where the default position about pain is the pain-relief paradigm and its result is the consequent cascade of medical interventions. These predictions are based on the likelihood (or not) of you being supported through crisis of confidence moments in birth settings dominated by a pain-relief mindset. In the present birth culture that likelihood is, of course, zilch.

Outcomes based on pain type

Pain-avoiding women

Remember, these women have their crisis of confidence before the labour. They are going to access pain relief, preferably an epidural on demand, probably in pre- or early labour, before they reach any physical distress. So they are knowingly, proactively jumping onto that cascade of interventions. They end up with high-intervention births and are generally satisfied with their experience. They are motivated to avoid the pain, and so as long as that happens, they are happy to accept the consequences.

'Status quo' women

These women generally hit a crisis at the shift between pre- and early labour (1–2 cm dilation)—the first of the predictable crises in the labour itself. Like the *pain-avoiding woman*, the *'status quo' woman* usually ends up with pain-relief options and a cascade birth, although by a more passive, acquiescent route than the clearly chosen route of the *pain-avoiding woman*. For the *'status quo' woman*, labour confirms their acculturated belief that birth is too painful and that they need saving by pain-relief options. These women come out of the birth with the belief that birth is too painful confirmed and so generally accept the inevitable cascade of interventions.

'Wait and see' women

These women have a sense that they can bring some capacity to work with their birthing body but they assume that they have a finite pain threshold. My prediction is that they will make it through the shift from pre- to early labour, but they are likely to be stumped by a crisis at the shift from early labour into established labour, somewhere around

4–6 cm dilation. They have waited, they have seen and they don't like! Then it's an easy slide down to the usual cascade of interventions being set in play via the pain-relief pathway. These women come out of the birth with a diminished sense of their stamina and capacity, which is not a great start for the fifty-plus years of mothering coming up.

'Aspirational but naïve' women

Because they have done a lot of preparation these women will generally rise to the escalating challenge and move through pre- to early labour, and then from early to established labour. But they get caught up *big time* at the 7 cm crisis of confidence. Then, with their self-belief crumbling and with no capacity to normalise and accept that it can feel this bad and still be okay, they begin the predictable slide into the interventions via the pain-relief pathways, too.

Psychologically, the *aspirational but naïve woman* comes out of the birth experience in worst shape. Because they expect to be able to rely on their own personal power and control, rather than seeing labour as a team effort, these women don't set up support they can lean into during this crisis of confidence. Of all the attitude groups, the *aspirational naïve woman* runs the greatest risk of feeling she has 'failed' when her aspiration for normal physiological birth is not realised. In some cases, this sense of personal failure may extend into post-natal depression. If you have understood what I am saying about the circles of influence on pain in labour, then rather than these women feeling they have failed, you might feel that our birth culture in fact has 'failed' them.

'Pain-embracing' women

Like the *aspirational but naïve woman*, the *pain-embracing woman* has put in the preparation work that carries her through till she hits the 7 cm crisis. But here's where they differ. For the *pain-embracing woman*, this is where her savvy understanding of the birth culture and a realistic take on pain and support needs will stand her in good stead. This awareness means she will have set up a *facilitating holding circle* that now draws in close, normalises her crisis and boosts her pain tolerance by enabling her to ride their waves of confidence in her ability.

These women generally fulfil their intention and yearning for a normal physiological birth. They are the women who come out of the birth with the feeling that 'with the right support I can do any bloody thing!' This is a brilliant way to start those fifty or more years of mothering ahead.

No guarantee

Of course, there are other factors that can have an impact on a birth's outcome. While being a major influence, pain types and pain dynamics are not the only factors that shape the outcome of a labour. Working through your attitudes and choices about pain can turn you towards a normal physiological birth, but it does not guarantee this outcome. There are times in some labours when true medical need situations arise and require interventions to keep the mother and baby safe, trumping any of these pain types and pain-dynamic considerations.

However, if there was a cultural shift and 'working with pain' became the dominant paradigm and 'working with pain' options were the default reality, all the circles of influence pressing onto the birthing woman would support 'working with pain' attitudes. Midwives and support circles would be on board with good 'working with pain' skills and the birthing woman at the centre of all that support wouldn't be left alone wrestling with her inner 'wimp demons', with only her own determination to try to see her through.

Then I believe many 'status quo', 'wait and see', and 'aspirational but naïve' women would be supported to work with pain and so make it through, enabling increasing numbers of mothers and babies to benefit from the advantages of normal physiological birth. (Pinch me, I must be dreaming!)

Conclusion

While these individual attitudes to pain have consequences, remember they are shaped by a particular social and cultural milieu. Nonetheless, if you are a willing woman with intentions towards a physiologically normal birth, then working out your personal pain attitude, checking its compatibility with your aspirations, and how it measures up against my predictions are crucial.

I've presented this mapping of the pathways predicted by pain types to many midwives and obstetricians over the years and they all agree that yes, 'that's exactly what happens'. This is also true in my experience with birthing women themselves. I've talked to many women having their second or third babies, who also say that this analysis of how their pain type meets the birth culture entirely explains what happened during the experience of their first birth.

I do hope you find this useful and that it will help you to make wise choices in support of your yearning. Because an understanding of your pain type and how it can influence your birth outcome will give you the best chance of making your way through one of the most crucial challenges of labour—a crisis of confidence.

Personal reflections

- Do you have a buffer zone provided by your wider circle of family and friends?
- Have you ensured a buffer zone by your choice of birth-place culture?
- How will your midwife know you are a willing woman?
- How will you know if your midwife is a 'working with pain' midwife?
- Do you have support for 'working with pain'?
- Are you organising a 'naïve support circle' or a 'facilitating holding circle'?
- What is your attitude to pain in labour?
- According to my predictions, how compatible is your attitude with your intentions?

5

Crisis of confidence: when self-belief crumbles

'I can't do it anymore … my back hurts, my back hurts so much. I didn't know it was going to be like this … if I could just get a little break … I just need a little break … Pleeeese, I need a break … get me something … Help me! Help me!'

This, or something like it, is the lament of the birthing woman in a crisis of confidence.

It's not as if most birthing women have an absolute trust and faith in themselves at the start of the labour that then continues as a smooth run through until the very end. No, that self-belief is challenged. In the first place, the birthing woman has to build her belief in her birthing capacity and in her 'working with pain' capacity against a backdrop of powerful negative cultural messages. Then, in the labour, she has to continually re-engage with that belief again and again. The building intensity of the labour creates peaks and pain 'edges', taking the birthing woman past her comfort zone and discomfort zone into pain and transformation zones—and each of these 'edges' can bring the potential for a 'crisis of confidence' to occur. During these crises of confidence, a birthing woman feels that she doesn't have the resources to match the intensity of the labour—the pain is too much, too strong, too tiring. It's all too overwhelming. She wants saving, she wants out, she wants drugs and she wants them now! Some years ago, in the *Weekend Australian*, Patrica Morey wrote this about her birth: 'Disillusioned and desperate, caught up in a process you are unable to control and drowning in waves of excruciating pain, you beg in turn for the gas mask, the pethidine, the epidural.'[56] This is the cry of the birthing woman in a crisis of confidence. She is swept up by birthing energies she can't control, taken to that edge. When a birthing woman, even a 'willing woman', is in the grip of this crisis of confidence she wants out—out of the work of it, out of the pain. She wants what the cultural messages tell her she should expect: to be comfortable.

Sarah's story

I coined the phrase a 'crisis of confidence' many years ago after supporting a particularly challenging birth. Sarah was expecting her first baby—a long-awaited baby girl—with her husband, ten years into their marriage. They had chosen to birth at a birth centre, intending to have a water birth. Sarah regularly attended my weekly pregnancy sessions and asked me to support her at the birth. I was called to Sarah's labour by the birth centre midwife, who excitedly informed me on the phone that I had better hurry if I wanted to make it, because Sarah was in transition and the baby would be here soon. Knowing Sarah's story, I had expected this to be a long, difficult labour, but according to the midwife my prediction was way off the mark. It seemed that after only a few hours of building labour Sarah was ready to push her baby out.

I had worked with this experienced midwife before, so I respected her assessment of the situation. Yet I felt an intuitive niggle that left me with some disquiet. When I arrived at the birth centre I found Sarah and her husband in the birth tub with the midwife watching on. As I sat with them through a few contractions, I could see why the midwife had assumed that the birth of the baby was close. Sarah was exhibiting the classic signs we interpret as 'transition'—intense contractions, emotional distress, complaining that she couldn't go on, pleading for relief and that it all needed to *stop now!* She also had a catch in her breath at the peak of the contractions, an indication that maybe she was ready to begin 'bearing down'.

Sarah's behaviour was certainly similar to transition-like expressions, but I wasn't convinced; it still didn't sound or feel quite right to me. In trying to resolve this discrepancy I asked the midwife if she had done a vaginal examination in order to confirm that the opening of Sarah's cervix was actually matching her outward expressions, and that she was really ready to move into active second-stage pushing. The midwife felt there was no need for an internal examination as the signs of transition and early second stage were clear. While I, too, generally see no need for routine vaginal examinations, in this situation I was still not fully convinced that the labour was as far advanced as it appeared. My intuitive niggle had grown stronger. So, after gaining permission from Sarah and asking for the midwife's support, the midwife performed a vaginal examination.

This revealed that, far from being in transition, Sarah was 2 cm dilated, in fact—she was still in pre-labour. For Sarah, this presented a major challenge. She lost her resolve and belief in her capacity and became dispirited and despairing about her ability or willingness to go on. However, her birth choices served her well here. Her carefully chosen birth team—her *facilitating holding circle*—supported Sarah to regroup. She returned home, where she said, 'this became a crying time, crying the grief of felt failure, confronting the fear of the unknowable to come'. Then, after spending time sleeping, resting, walking, crying and grieving, Sarah's contractions, after having slowed, built again. She eventually returned to the birth centre, where, with intense support, she continued—rocking, dancing and working with her labour. Finally Sarah, as she had intended, triumphantly birthed her baby girl in that same birth tub some twenty-four hours later.

'Crisis of confidence' versus 'transition'

Sarah's birth experience confirmed for me that a woman in labour could exhibit strong expressions of distress, which might resemble what we would usually understand as 'transition', but which were not.

Reflecting on this birth with the midwife, I could see that the discrepancy between Sarah's behaviour and the assessment that she was 2 cm dilated had been a surprise to the midwife. But if Sarah's experience of emotional distress and intense contractions wasn't transition, what was it?

Sarah's experience is what I have now come to call a 'crisis of confidence' in particular, a 2 cm 'anxiety crisis'—an exaggerated pain response fuelled by anxiety. When women experiencing this crisis are supported and able to connect with the reality of their body rather than with the 'freak out' of their anxiety, they can steady themselves. The experience of their contractions settles and their behaviour more accurately reflects what is actually physiologically happening in their bodies.

Unfortunately, what can happen instead is that a crisis of confidence is misinterpreted, with big impacts on the birth—as Tania's story, told to me by another birth attendant, illustrates.

Tania's story

The birth attendant, who had trained with me, explained that she had been working with Tania, a first-time mother, whose contractions had grown stronger.

Tania was having trouble getting into a rhythm and started to complain that she couldn't go on much longer and that it was too painful. To the birth attendant, it seemed that Tania was having a 'crisis of confidence', but the attending midwife again seemed to think that she was going through transition and had started asking her if she had an urge to push.

Tania was confused. All she knew was that it was intense. Because her legs were shaking, she accepted the midwife's suggestion that she have a sit on the birth stool and try some pushing. The birth attendant told me:

> I didn't feel like we were up to the pushing stage yet, even after thirty minutes or so of attempts at pushing. So I suggested that she might want to have an internal to see what she was up to. Tania wasn't fully dilated at all, but was at 7 cm. She broke down at this point and there was no consoling her, the devastation of thinking she was nearly there and then discovering that she wasn't, proved impossible to recover from. She decided to have an epidural, which then set in motion the predictable cascade of interventions resulting in an episiotomy and vacuum extraction.

Crisis of confidence: the challenging edge of achievement

Before my experience of Sarah's birth, I used to describe experiences of panic and distress such as hers as an indication of a 'place of challenge'[57] that was likely to confront women carrying particular distressing life experiences into their births.

However, in talking about this misinterpreted 'crisis' dynamic more widely with women and midwives, I came to see that it was also occurring in labours where no such previous distressing life experiences existed. So, as an educator, I began to describe this experience as a 'crisis of confidence' rather than a particular 'place of challenge', in order to cover not only distress and resistance arising from difficult life stories, but also the more usual crises of confidence arising simply from the physical demands of the labour.

For me, this concept of 'crisis of confidence' had a quality that was familiar. I was reminded of my years as a physical education and outdoor adventure teacher, during which I had witnessed that many of us, when confronted by challenging physical demands, can crumble mentally and emotionally—and consequently not realise our true physical capacity for achievement. I was also reminded of my counselling work and recognised the resistant distress that can manifest in counselling sessions when difficult emotional material is awakened and requires processing. In fact, when you start to think about it, I'm sure you, too, can recognise this concept of a 'crisis of confidence' in many areas of life.

Physical pain crisis

A physiologically driven loss of self-belief in the face of intense functional demand is probably the most common pathway to a crisis of confidence in labour, but it is not, of course, confined to birthing. It is found on netball courts, soccer fields and football grounds, gym circuit classes, weights rooms, swimming pools, bike tracks, dance and yoga studios. It's found anywhere people are undertaking challenging physical activities. Joggers in parks and bike riders up hills experience it; bushwalkers carrying heavy packs know it well, as do rock and mountain climbers, circus performers and all manner of endurance enthusiasts. I, in recent years, have come to engage with it again in marathon kayaking and have known it far too intimately at many points on the long paddles! Within this domain of physically demanding experiences, whether for fitness, endurance, peak performance or personal-best achievement, the experience of a crisis of confidence is akin to the range of challenges we call 'hitting the wall', 'going to the next level', 'breaking through the pain barrier', approaching 'the hurt zone', needing to 'dig deep', 'answering the question', and many more. These challenges are an expected and prepared-for test of capacity, stamina, determination and courage.

Over the years, for various presentations, I have interviewed women who embrace physically demanding effort for achievement. I asked these women if they experienced moments during their achievements when they were filled with self-doubt and didn't feel that they could go on. 'Of course,' said marathon swimmer Tammy van Wisse. Circus performer Andrea agreed: 'Everybody gets to a point of wanting to give up.'[58]

These women accepted that in their strong physical endeavours, even with preparation, these crisis points would occur. Their strategies for working through these crises included seeking support, using pre-organised inspirational key words and phrases, visualisation, focusing on regaining rhythm and, above all, remembering that these crises were *an expected part of the process.*

Psychological pain crisis

As well as crises sparked by physiological pain, there is, of course, the related challenge of emotional and psychological pain. Again, it's worth remembering that we face these challenges in many domains. 'Crises of confidence' can arise from the emotional and psychological challenges faced by people working in the creative arts, or studying for educational achievements, or working through psychological pain or spiritual distress.

Creative artists of all types willingly enter their work with the knowledge that psychologically based 'crises of confidence' will be part of their journey.

In fact, many creative people *revere* these unsettling, disorganised, vulnerable, 'not knowing how to go on' moments, and honour them as episodes of 'divine perturbation'. They recognise them as times when their self-doubts are up and their psyche is working overtime, making ready for a creative outpouring to come.

James Guppy, an artist and artist retreat facilitator, speaking on Radio National's *Art Works* (26 June 2011), mentioned that artists go through strong distressing emotions, usually when they are on the verge of a breakthrough in their work.[59]

In a series of interviews I did with various creative artists for a conference presentation[60], writer Joanna Murray-Smith also spoke of emotionally painful times in her writing process and drew parallels with her birth experiences:

> Once you accept that you are a writer you recognise that you often get taken to a very dark emotional place, certainly a very frightening emotional place, because it's not controlled. I mean, it can be exhilarating as well, but … even when it's seemingly positive, it's still frightening because it's not controlled. I always know that I'm going to be mining parts of myself, which are almost certainly going to be uncomfortable. And if the intensity doesn't happen then the whole experience is compromised. I suppose it makes for a wearying life. But it's exciting; it is exciting. So it is in birth, in my births.

Joanna then goes on to describe a common experience of self-doubt manifesting in a crisis of confidence about her writing:

> Well I think that doubting voice is there all the time. The more deeply we investigate the weirdness of the self in the process of writing, the more that defeating voice is present, because you find all the time you are looking for a way out! You are looking for a way to avoid that painful experience.

In an article in the *Age* (15 October 2011) novelist Alex Miller also reiterated Joanna's point when he wrote: 'every book has a point of crisis it must survive; every book has a moment when it appears impossible'.[61]

Well-known film director Jane Campion, in a magazine interview for *The Good Weekend* magazine (5 December, 2009), also colourfully describes a crisis of confidence process in her creative work: 'I'd feel like there were voices in my mind going, 'You're f… ing pathetic. You're hopeless'. This is the sort of dialogue I live with. My unconscious would get going before I'd even have a chance to say, 'Stop'. It'd be, 'You're a joke. You're full of shit'. Then I'd go, 'Grrr', and struggle my way into the day.'[62]

In her interview with me[63], actor Eugenia Fragos develops this theme further:

> You know you are going to have to go somewhere dark. I can feel that building and I can go into rehearsal feeling, 'Oh my god is it going to be today? No, I'm not ready, I'm not psychically ready to go there'. Often the worst performance would come just before you were about to make another breakthrough, because the ground had shifted again and you were holding onto how it was the first two or three performances. Now it's starting to unravel, because the work was starting to go deeper and you're kind of resisting that because you've just hit a comfort zone with it. You don't want to friggin change it again! But the work calls it from you and demands: the text, your fellow actors, the piece itself has an entity and that demands that it keeps changing—but you resist that.

Isn't that a brilliant description? Eugenia's experience shares such similarities with the resistant 'crisis of confidence' process that birthing women struggle through. In our interview[64] Andrew Bovell, playwright, dramaturge and writer, perhaps most widely known for the film *Lantana*, added to the theme:

> There are big blocks and little blocks. The big blocks are about self-esteem, self-belief. When you get over those, then there are blocks within the work. It's relentless. But there are points in the work where I lose it. I lose my capacity to believe in myself that I can do it.

I am invariably reminded of this crisis of confidence dynamic playing out with predictable regularity when I reflect on the process of supporting family members and friends through educational and academic achievements. If you have been close to anyone completing their HSC, VCE or a Masters or PhD thesis, you will no doubt have witnessed many crises of confidence. In this context at least, you will also hopefully have recognised these crisis moments as the challenging edge of achievement.

We face crises of confidence in so many areas of our lives and often, even though we don't like them, we nonetheless understand them as challenging processes of growth. If we frame it at an existential level, any crisis of confidence can become a place of meaning, if witnessed, honoured and supported for the transformative potential it offers.

Richness of life experiences

'Crisis of confidence' experiences seem to be par for the course in most challenging creative and intellectual endeavours, just as they are in physical peak-performance achievements. I'm pretty sure we all know this about difficult achievements in life, but somehow we can't accept it in birthing. Just reflect for a moment on what might happen to any artist's work—Joanna and Alex's novels and plays, Eugenia's performances, Andrew's writing or Jane's films—if they, in the midst of their crises of confidence, had their self-doubting limitations confirmed by their publishers, directors, financial backers or audiences. If they received agreement that, in fact, they couldn't do it, and that, yes, it was too much for them (after all they don't have to be martyrs to their art do they?). Do we imagine that human culture throughout time would have had the richness of the expressive arts that, as actor Eugenia says 'at its best is transformative and has the power to touch a person's soul', without artists being supported through these crises? Luckily, these artists and writers and performers *are* supported. Joanna Murray-Smith explains:

> When I'm in a crisis, I say to my publisher, 'I can't finish the book'. And they say, 'Of course you can and you will because you're a great writer and the last [book] was fantastic. Remember how difficult that was and look at the way it turned out'.

What would happen to any deeply affecting works of art or scholarship or spiritual insight, if the artist or scholar, in their crisis of confidence, were *not* supported through?

We might ponder what richness of human spirit and connectedness we, as individual women and as a community, and our children, are deprived of when we deny birthing women the safe space and attuned support necessary to work with and through any crises of confidence they experience in their labours.

Imagine this. A birthing woman; she's on a groove, she's working with her contractions—breathing, moving, rocking, releasing. Yes! Beautiful! Yes, she can do it! Then it all ramps up, her contractions build—stronger, longer, deeper, closer together—just as they should, going up through the gears, revving harder and stronger, doing the work, opening her body. But she doesn't like it. Doesn't like being dragged out of her comfort zone, through her discomfort zone and way out into her pain zone. Or she feels she's already used all her best moves; or she's unprepared for the ramp-up; or she's fearful of how much longer it will take, especially if she feels she's only just keeping it together now and it's still getting stronger. Her positive self-talk crumbles, all her carefully constructed images, affirmations, intentions, breathing and relaxation practices are out the window, replaced, at first, by pleading, whinging, crying, and later by ranting and finally the crescendo of the contemporary birthing woman's much-heard mantra—'get me the fucking epidural!'

The birthing woman cries out for 'help' at these 'crisis of confidence' moments, exposing her vulnerability as she faces a struggle that touches the core of her self-belief. How will she be met in this vulnerability and neediness?

This is where 'pain dynamics' get underway. And these dynamics mean the outcome, at the time of a crisis of confidence, is more in the hands of the support that surrounds her, or not, than within the birthing woman herself. What happens at this point is actually up to who is supporting her and what they are going to do about it. Because if it's left to the birthing woman now, it's a done deal—breathing is out, and drugs or an epidural are in.

Support for achievement

The story of Sarah's birth deepened my awareness about emotional distress in labour and was an inspirational story for me. However, I was mindful that her birth experience could just as easily not have unfolded in the ultimately satisfying way it did.

If Sarah, who had also thought she was in 'transition' at 2 cm dilation, had not been in a care setting where she received the support needed to regroup and work through this crisis, I have no doubt her birth experience would have headed down the more usual pathway of the cascade of interventions.

For the willing woman, with her yearning towards normal physiological birth, this issue of preparing for, recognising and then working through any crises of confidence becomes vital.

'Helping' in the labour-bypass era

In this present labour-bypass era, what does 'help' for birthing women look like? What support is given to the birthing woman in her struggle, in her 'crisis of confidence?' What answer to her self-doubt is offered? Birthing women are pitied as victims of their birthing bodies and this pity is at its greatest when they are in the throes of a crisis of confidence. 'The poor things, it's too much for them, they shouldn't have to suffer' is the dominant attitude. Wanting to rescue women from the painful, effort-filled work of labour is the common response, which only confirms the birthing woman's lack of capacity in her own mind.

This is a betrayal. And a doubly cruel wounding often occurs around this betrayal when, after the birth, many mothers come to feel that the very drugs or epidural offered them in their moment of crisis are a proof of her personal failure. Shame, guilt and personal blame abound. Patricia Morey, in the newspaper article mentioned earlier, continues: 'In the depths of despair you know that you've blown the birth and in doing so you've failed the first test of motherhood.'[65]

I know it can be different. I know that every woman has a deeper intention and continuity, even if, in the present moments of crisis, that deeper intention seems to be missing. If she can be guided into a renewed rhythm of engagement with her labour, the birthing woman can be supported to rise from the vulnerability of a crisis of confidence and, like a phoenix from the ashes, open into expanded resourcefulness. Michelle G experienced a crisis of confidence with her first baby and her story illustrates the kind of 'help' a *facilitating* birth team can provide.

Michelle's story

After some time in early labour Michelle G moved into established labour at around 4 cm dilation.

> My contractions were much stronger and regular and I was very proud of how I was handling the pain. Moving, squatting and breathing just like the women in the active birth videos who look so beautiful and empowered.

Several hours later she was in intense labour, in the birthing tub, and surrounded by her midwife, two experienced women friends and me. She remembers:

> I had forgotten my romantic images and was kneeling in the tub howling from the depths of my soul, convinced that the pain was too much to bear.

At this time of crisis her partner and mother, finding the emotional intensity too confronting, had retreated to the garden, while her support circle of experienced women drew closer, offering guidance and expressing belief in her capacity to go on. Michelle G continues:

> Not that I got any sympathy … instead, I was showered with reassurance, love and incredible strength from the energy and wise words of those who were present to witness and support. I was surrounded by such powerful women: all mothers who I loved and admired. They showed me strengths I never realised I possessed. Then later, my baby started on the final phase of her journey. The burning was so intense, the pushing unbelievable, wonderful, and all I wanted was for her to come out. I needed her to know how much I longed to hold her, so I kept calling to her silently at first and then louder and louder, 'Come on baby, come on!' and suddenly there she was … my little girl.

Disorganised moments

Even a willing woman, strong in her own birth power, will be challenged at predictable points during the labour. At moments of surging hormones and intensifying contractions, women can become momentarily disorganised. What they've been doing in the labour so far is no longer enough to match the ramp-up in intensity. So what now? 'Can I?' the woman ponders. She might fall momentarily into thinking, 'I don't think I can' or 'I don't want to' or 'I shouldn't have to' or '*I bloody well won't*'.

If the birthing woman can't match, or isn't supported to match, this increased intensity—this necessary, building functional pain—then this momentary disorganisation can deteriorate into a panic state, which then can develop into a full-blown crisis of confidence. Especially if she feels she is already at the end of her tether and struggling to cope: then her fears and self-doubts, amplified by the pain-relief birth culture, spread like wildfire in her psyche.

The research into 'flow' states can help us understand something of what's going on here. To achieve a flow state a delicate balance between skills and challenges is required. If skills exceed challenges, we relax but eventually become bored, which may pose a problem in pre- and early labour. However, if distractions disrupt the experience, or challenges exceed skills, we become vigilant and then anxious, setting up the conditions for a crisis of confidence to develop. Most birthing women, especially in a first labour, irrespective of their intentions beforehand and even if they have diligently prepared, still come up against these crises—and there can be more than one in a powerfully developing labour.

Medical crisis versus crisis of confidence

Before I describe this crisis of confidence phenomenon any further, it's important to be clear about what I do and do not mean here. When I use the term 'crisis of confidence' I am *not* speaking about a medical, 'things going wrong' crisis. I am speaking about a distress response to the intensity of the functional pain of normal birth—a state of emotional turmoil, hitting a pain barrier, in which the mother's usual coping strategies and even her well-practised birth skills seem no match for what she is facing. This crisis is not a sign that anything is *going wrong*. Far from it. In fact, it is usually a sign that *everything is going brilliantly!* If this is understood and women are well supported, then these crises usually don't last long. However, these crisis moments are *critical*, pivotal moments, because the way they are resolved will affect the further course of the labour.

In terms of the willing woman's original yearning towards normal birth, things will either get better or worse from here. The quality of support is crucial. Does she have anybody who knows how to encourage her, anyone who can contain her vulnerability and anxiety? Anyone who can help her regain her rhythm? Does she have anyone who can sweet-talk her back into her strength, anyone who can drag her, kicking and complaining, across her own imagined limitations and resistance and on into her birthing power? Or is she surrounded by people who want to 'save' her from the painful work of it? We'll discuss these support issues in the next chapter. For now, let me give you more of an idea of *when* and *why* women experience a crisis of confidence.

Predictable crisis of confidence points in labour

I've found that there are some predictable times in labour where these crises of confidence usually occur, activated (in the main) by the intensifying hormonal surges that create the potent, deeper, longer, stronger and closer-together contractions that drive the birth process. Crises of confidence occur at those points when the labour shifts gear—it's all revving harder and birthing women have to shift their gear ratio to match the greater demand.

Crisis of 'culture calling'

Increasingly, more women are experiencing their first crisis of confidence—what I call the crisis of 'culture calling'—before they're even in labour. This is an 'anticipatory' crisis. Acculturated fears about pain and danger coupled with socially conditioned 'pain relief' attitudes toward controlling or eliminating labour pain, lead to this crisis. This crisis underpins the pain-avoiding attitude referred to in the previous chapter.

Crisis of 'mind calling'

The next crisis may be experienced at about 1–2 cm dilation at the shift from pre- to early labour. I've come to call this one the crisis of 'mind calling'. This is the 'anxiety' crisis. The mother's thinking, worrying brain is still active and may be filled with anxieties and fears about the birth, baby, or the coming life changes. Resistant energy is now in the mix, increasing physical pain through the 'fear-tension-pain' response—that is, fear causes a release of adrenalin that, in addition to other effects, causes elevated muscle tension that then ramps up the pain level. *Status quo women* often get diverted down the intervention pathway at this crisis point.

Crisis of 'the body calling'

The next shift in intensity, which marks the progression from early labour to established labour (sometimes also known as active labour) at around 4–6 cm dilation, provides the next likely crisis—the crisis of 'the body calling'. This is the woman's challenge of committing to the *embodiment* of labour. The challenge of committing to feeling her body working. Can she stay with the experience of her body? She wants the baby, but does she want to feel her body working? Does she want to engage with the functional pain? How much stronger and longer is it going to be? This point is the test of the *wait and see woman*'s pain threshold.

Crisis of 'evolution calling'

Another shift in hormones, experienced around 7 cm dilation, drives another major crisis—the crisis of 'evolution calling'. This is an 'overwhelm' crisis. At this stage, the shift in consciousness orchestrated by the endorphins is really driving the evolutionary regression outlined in chapter 3. Everything is driven by an urgency and intensity that is becoming impossible to control.

Does the labouring woman trust the birthing process with its evolutionary script enough to surrender to it? Does she feel safe enough? Can she surrender ego-control and allow this shift in consciousness, this evolutionary regression, to release primal birthing woman? Can she hold a centre in the midst of these storms of labour? Here we have the 'overwhelm' crisis that often separates the *aspirational but naïve woman* from the *pain-embracing woman*.

Transition

Then, of course, the more familiar 'transition' occurs (8–10 cm dilation), when the completion of the opening of the woman's cervix and the transitioning energy in her body—from 'drawing up' to 'bearing down'—occurs creating confusion and distress.

Crisis of 'baby calling'

For some women, there may also be the crisis of 'baby calling' in second stage when the stretch receptors, activated on the perineum, create the outrageous intensity commonly referred to as the 'ring of fire'. This physical intensity itself can cause a resistant crisis but also exacerbate any *unresolved resistance to change*. Is the birthing woman and her life situation ready to receive her baby?

Stages of labour and hormonal surges (Fig 5.1)

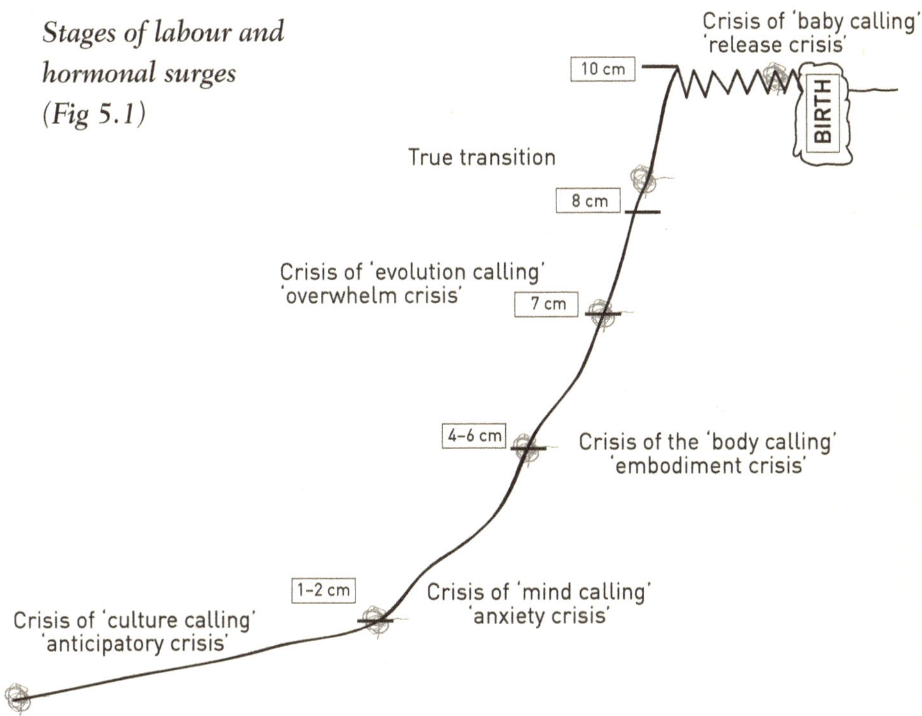

Realistic expectations

Let me be clear: the issue is not so much *whether* a crisis will develop—but what is going to happen *when* it occurs.

Returning to the artistic sphere, we can see that *expecting* this crisis of confidence can be helpful. I asked Jenny Kemp, a playwright and theatre director, what she does when she hits a crisis in her work.[66]

> What do I do? It probably happens in every process, losing the plot at some point, saying 'I can't do this'. When it happens I now say to myself— 'Jenny, this is rather familiar'. It doesn't mean that I don't completely lose the plot and get into black depressions and think what I'm doing is a pile of shit; it doesn't mean any of that doesn't happen. Just that these are the ways that I negotiate my way through it.

'So it's normalising these crises of confidence rather than seeing them as something abnormal?' I ask. *'Yes, yes, yes,'* she replies.

Remember the mantra I repeat in my birth preparation workshops, 'you don't have to like it to do it brilliantly'?—well the following story from a colleague, who describes supporting a mother through the full range of dramatic crises of confidence, certainly proves my point.

Julie's story

Julie was in early labour when she hit the 1–2 cm anxiety crisis. The birth attendant recalls:

> She looked at me slightly exasperated but with great sincerity and said 'I don't think I can do this!' I could hear in her voice that Julie's resistance was high and she would start to chant 'No, no, no!' as a contraction took hold. Later on in the labour, Julie would become an angry, frustrated 'toddler-teenager', but here she reverted into 'sobbing, helpless, little-girl' mode.

The established labour, the 'crisis of the body calling' of 4–6 cm saw her sobbing and pleading for it all to stop, then relaxing as she collapsed into her partner's chest and sobbed. At 7 cm the 'overwhelm' crisis of intense labour kicked in.

> She started raging and demanding 'drugs!', wanting an epidural, or better still, a caesarean section so that she could just be knocked out. She was becoming quite angry and abusive. Julie

> was convinced now that an epidural would be the only thing that would help her.

Finally, at true transition:

> Julie demanded she be allowed to leave because she wasn't going to do this anymore! 'Just kill me'. And began ranting and raving again about how, if it was like this now she couldn't possibly go through 'transition'. John [her partner] and Julie built up to this emotional climax with one another and she slapped him.

Julie's labour ended an hour or so later with the exhilarating birth of a healthy, cuddly boy, without any recourse to pain relief. She had the attuned intense support from her partner, birth attendant, and hospital midwife helping her through these crises of confidence, as well as the more steady, focused, 'flow state' hours of labouring that came between each of these dramatic, zone-edge crises. Julie's was a demanding but straightforward normal physiological birth. If this description is confronting, that's okay, because for the willing woman, having realistic expectations about these crises is important. Having realistic expectations can galvanise you to develop internal resources, as well as to seek experienced support to back your intentions. Samara recalls:

> The 'crisis of confidence' happened at the expected times: 3 cm dilated, when I was asking for pethidine, then later as well, before transition. Thank god my birth team had been to your workshop so they knew how to keep me going.

For the willing woman it's far better to be real than to be surprised or shocked by the intensity, and then left with nowhere to go but down the drug, epidural and 'cascade of interventions' pathways. Realistic expectations—rather than either exaggerated fears or naïvely romantic ideals that leave you unprepared for the hard work—better serve your capacity for birthing. And if it's not as challenging or painful as you expect? Well then, you'll be laughing!

Physiological demand

Because the pathway to crisis involves physical pain, let me say again, by pain here I am referring to *physiological* pain: the metabolic physiological demand, felt in a healthy body working well but at levels of high intensity, beyond usual comfort levels. I am not referring to pain that comes from disease, damage or injury—*pathological* pain. I've touched on some of these 'why' issues in earlier chapters, but want to tease out some more themes in the context of this crisis of confidence.

Our current lifestyle does not, in the main, support birthing women. Generally, we've become a sedentary, comfort-seeking people. We are no longer, as a matter of need, required to experience our body's strength, stamina, or straining effort, or required on a daily basis to keep persevering through bodily experiences of discomfort, stretch, strain, functional pain or complex movement—the great variety of movements that once gave a natural outlet for our bodies to strengthen and function at their full potential. As Linda Hartley observes in *Wisdom of the Body Moving*: 'The advancement of industrial and technological cultures have also separated us more and more from the earth and the free movement of our bodies. Most of us today, perform within only a very limited range of the movements that our bodies are capable of undertaking. This can cause a gradual stagnation of energy and loss of expression, vitality and awareness.'[67]

We are not served well by our culture and lifestyle to be able to normalise—as healthy and positive—a continuum of bodily experience ranging from discomfort through to intensely painful effort. Unless we actively choose to engage with demanding body experiences, outside of a narrow comfort zone, we are left with a severely diminished pain tolerance. For a contemporary birthing woman whose baseline experience of her body's capacity for engagement with powerful striving effort is minimal, the work of labouring takes her on a hyper-leap into outer space, way past her existing comfort zones and bodily experience. Once, when we experienced in our daily life the need for a range of sweating, straining, tiring physical actions, the birthing experience of early and active labour had a reference point akin to that of other normal, functional demanding efforts. Back then, 'transition'—the difficult period of late first-stage labour—was the typical challenge point where crisis behaviours surfaced. Now, due to this societal shift to a largely sedentary and physically 'comfortable' lifestyle, and with the seductive epidural escape clause, we find birthing women already struggling and distressed at much earlier points in the labour.

Remember in chapter 3, when I discussed the fact that we all appear to have a 'pain-killer' mindset? Well, added to this is the effect on birth-pain tolerance of our socially encouraged medications for all menstrual discomforts—along with the added injunction to not in any way be inconvenienced by 'that time of the month'. Also, the widespread use of 'the pill'—offering us the possibility of controlling, not only our choices with regard to fertility, but also our menstrual rhythms—adds to this ingrained assumption that, along with targeted painkillers, we can be saved from any inconvenience, discomfort or pain we might feel as we open our bodies to bleed.

I know they are not still being packaged in this way but some years ago Panadol and Libra Fleur tampons had a *Trusted Partners Bonus Pack* in the supermarkets. The blurb on the pack said it all: 'Putting up with the pain and discomfort associated with menstruation, such as stomach cramping and back pain, can be frustrating and stressful. Panadol will quickly, simply and effectively manage your pain and allow you to confidently get on with your day.' Well if the message is that you *need* Panadol to 'manage' your menstrual pain you're definitely set up to *need* an epidural to 'manage' your labour pain. The advent of the pill and targeted pain relief, is of course positive in many ways, nonetheless it is limiting of women's resourcefulness, trust and capacity to normalise the functional pain of their birthing bodies.

Also, as I've said before, in labour the implications of this lack of a lived reality with functional, physiological pain, is compounded by the ready availability of epidural anesthesia. Even if a willing woman is intending, at the onset of her labour, to work with her pain, when the experience becomes arduous, and the ingrained cultural attitude of 'killing pain' takes over, the possibility of an epidural quickly dissolves the firm ground of her earlier resolve.

Sally, while preparing for the birth of her first baby, experienced an 'ah-ha' moment about her previous patterns with functional pain that helped her to prepare for any crisis of confidence moments in labour.

Sally's story

Sally and her partner had attended my birth preparation workshop and had received a paper I had written based on the interview I'd done with marathon swimmer Tammy van Wisse. Sally explains:

> The piece resonated with me. When I analysed my relationship with pain in swimming I realised that I always copped out. When I reached a crisis point, I crumbled, because at that moment when I doubted my ability to withstand the pain, I always found a justification for giving up. When I was younger I loved training—and at training I was as good as people who competed at a far higher level than myself—but I hated competition. I was not intellectually committed to it as a form of human behaviour. So when I reached that crisis point in competition, I had an easy way out. I just told myself that the competition was arbitrary. It was something I had brought on myself, and I wasn't doing it for anyone but myself. Therefore, it wasn't necessary for me to push myself beyond the pain in the way that other people seemed to do.
>
> My baby gave me a reason to find out if I could get past the crisis point. I wanted to give her the best entry to the world that I could. I didn't want her little system to have to deal with drugs. I also wanted to be present for the whole experience. I am proud of having a strong body. I didn't want to reduce my ability to use that strength by limiting my capacity to feel my body working. And I wanted to be fully cognisant of the experience; both for her, so that I could share her entry into the world, and for me, so I could finally experience pushing past that crisis point. I designed training sessions that I thought would help prepare me. I concentrated

> on swimming uncomfortable in-between distances. I worked on increasing my stamina with long sets and I swam a lot of 75 m sets, which I calculated took about as long as a really long contraction.

The preparations of Sally and her support team served her beautifully in the long, demanding labour of that first baby. She passed through many crises of confidence, but in each case she was supported into her fullest capacity. She continues:

> By around 9 am I was in tears. I went and had a bath and a really good sob. It was a full-body, wailing kind of sob that could be heard throughout most of the fifth floor of the hospital. It was the first time that I seriously thought about drugs. I didn't even bother to raise it with my partner, because I knew he was too well trained. I imagined a frustrating argument with him and my friend, where I insisted that I knew that I had said no to drugs under any 'normal' circumstances, except in case of a medical emergency, but now I really wanted them. And I imagined them going through the well-planned rigmarole of empathetically informing me just how strong I was, and how brilliantly I was doing, and just how much I didn't need the drugs, and I knew I would lose the argument. Although I felt like a rat trapped in a maze of my own making at the time, it was absolutely what I needed. I found that I felt much restored, and the cry had been a fantastic release.

Another crisis threatened to undermine Sally's capacity to continue with the hard work of the labour:

> At around 4 pm my mother popped her head through the door. As soon as my mother saw me in pain she burst into tears and said 'Oh, my little Sally'. It was the first time anyone had given me any real kind of sympathy. I could feel tears well behind my eyes and I knew that I had to get her out of the room. The possibility of being offered real 'sympathetic' comfort, rather than just resolved support, was too much for me.

Then, as Sally's long, demanding journey reached its climax, the potent and exhilarating experience of her baby daughter's birth was everything she had yearned, prepared and strived for:

> I felt each contraction roaring through my body. They seemed to come from somewhere in the earth and rip through me, vibrating as they went. It was like being in huge surf. You feel the wave coming from behind, rumbling along, and you know that unless you go with it, you're going to get pummeled. As each contraction or wave powered through me I yelled. Not a 'god this hurts' yell, but a yell full of power. As soon as Lucy was born, we snuggled her close … we held her in our arms and kissed and admired her.

Psychological processes

The particular patterned emotional ways we respond when confronted with hard 'stuff' in our lives—the self-talk, self-belief, dedicated focus, approach or avoidance strategies, or sabotage techniques we use—can all manifest in our births. In Claire's description of an early crisis she charts her particular pattern: self-pity then looking to be saved, then her determination kicks in:

> For a while I felt very sorry for myself and kept looking pleadingly at Paul, Deb and Raz—they kept saying 'You're doing so well', 'You're fantastic …' I thought, 'Who are they talking about? I'm clearly doing crap'. That desperate feeling didn't last long and I talked myself into 'hardening the fuck up'.

Who might we meet, on the testing ground of birthing—the 'little girl', the 'pleaser', the 'princess', the 'damsel in distress', the 'inner martyr', the 'inner judge', the 'inner wimp', the 'control freak', the 'victim' or, preferably, the 'warrior woman', the 'instinctive primal birth-giver', the 'birthing goddess'?

Marissa's story

Marissa was a willing woman birthing in a hospital where she was able to make a relationship with a 'known midwife'.

Marissa had good self-awareness about the patterns that would be problematic for her in labour, so she detailed the following points on her birth plan:

> Do not show me one ounce of sympathy during labour. I am a 'princess' and will seize upon any sympathy if I can. I need to be motivated in a strong and positive manner. I do not respond well to wishy-washy 'Come on, you can do it' chitchat. Tell me I am doing it! Show me how to do it! I really like to have a good cry sometimes so just let me. I find crying a great release. It doesn't mean that I am not coping.

After the birth of her big baby boy, she wrote her birth story and in it detailed her first crisis of confidence in early labour (1–2 cm).

> Frustration began to well up in me, I began to lose my confidence. Was I in labour yet? Aside from the five-minutely contractions I wasn't getting anything much else. By 4.30 am I cracked it, I felt sorry for myself. I pulled off the TENS machine and had a tantrum. I wanted to get into the bath to soothe my body. I wanted to sleep. I wanted reassurance. I wanted love. I wanted my baby out *now*!

With encouragement from her partner and midwife to move through this early emotional distress, Marissa eventually, after twenty hours of off-and-on, pre- and early labour, and eight hours of established labour, gave birth to her son in her own power and potency, just as she had intended. Marissa describes his birth:

> The baby inched out with each contraction slowly, slowly. Dan, my husband, had tears in his eyes when he announced that he could see the baby's little eyes and ears. That brought a huge smile to my face, my fears of tearing slipped away and I was overcome

> with sheer excitement. So I waited and at the beginning of the contraction I took in a deep breath, and on the release I pushed and bore down, visualising that breath pushing down from my head to my vagina. I let out a heaving, guttural moan. My midwife lifted the baby up into my arms, I twisted around on my knees, Dan was by the bed; I kissed him. I kept saying thank you and I love you; I was so filled with emotion.

Jo's story

Jo, another willing woman preparing for her first birth, presented her homebirth caregivers with a birth plan that included self-awareness around this issue of crisis of confidence:

> When I ask for drugs I do not mean it. In this scenario, do two things: encourage me to change my scenery and leave me alone to wail for a few minutes (the baby's room is most probably the best place for me). After I've hit rock bottom, I will turn into Mr Hyde and want to be proactive. During this time, I would like you to help me to continue active birth positions.

After a crisis of confidence as she moved into established labour (4–6 cm), which her support circle—using this awareness of Jo's patterns—enabled her to work through, Jo birthed her baby in her cosy lounge room. She describes his welcome in a letter to her new baby:

> Daddy was walking around the lounge room with you in his arms—it was the most perfect moment. Within twenty minutes, I had cleaned up and was sitting on the couch in my PJs with a glass of champagne in hand. I felt like I had just run a marathon—alive, thrilled and exhausted all at the same time. We started breastfeeding immediately, while Daddy prepared Vietnamese chicken and corn soup for us all to feast on.

Cathartic release

Another dynamic that can link to a crisis of confidence is the experience of cathartic release. Many of us, maybe more usually women than men, have experienced first-hand (particularly when we are feeling emotionally overloaded) the immense relief of pent-up feelings, frustrations or anguished misery that a 'good cry' provides. In labour there can be many instances where crises of confidence trigger this type of emotional release. They can work wonders, enabling birthing women to let go of present or old 'stuff'. As Trish, referring to the birth experience of her first baby, so vividly puts it:

> I'd never felt so justified in having a good yell. This was my child's gift to me: the chance to finally throw it all out, my pain collection, old and musty, out and gone to the gods, never to return. Ahhhhhh … bellowing never felt so good.

In these situations, once again, the response of those surrounding the birthing woman will be crucial to what's going to happen in the labour. Can the support circle normalise and contain any cathartic release? Or do the support people and caregivers become fearful, distressed or even embarrassed, and therefore want to suppress the emotional release? If they do the latter it's a pity, because so often it feels good to the birthing woman and creates a way forward for the birth. As psychotherapist Professor Eugene Gendlin says: 'Catharsis of negative affect [emotions] feels good when it rolls out from the person, but painful when it comes at an observer who is not familiar with it.'[68]

Of course, for a support person to recognise this as positive relies very much on an experienced discernment. Also for the birthing woman herself, because even though a cathartic release may be excellent for progress in labour, without good support she may be left feeling embarrassed or ashamed of her outburst.

I remember being with May during her homebirth when her labour stalled. She explained later that she had always felt that she had been stuck in a pattern of being a 'good little girl' endlessly trying to please others. She described as exhilarating and transformational the liberation she felt when her frustration at the stalled energy and impasse in her labour was eventually unleashed as a full-blown cathartic temper tantrum in her bath—flailing and splashing water everywhere as she ranted and raved and yelled and cursed, demanding to go to hospital to get some drugs, and be saved from all the pain. Not least, she said, because she felt completely safe to do it, safely surrounded by her support people (who, I must say were all crowded in the far corner of the bathroom attempting to remain dry, yet delighting in witnessing this cathartic expression and the consequent unblocking of the stalled energy in her labour). No one was fearful, no one offended, there was no one 'to please' and definitely no one giving into May's demands to be 'saved'. A safe emotional container was provided—a 'holding circle'—allowing a powerful release that enabled May to move through this crisis and on into the developing intensity of her labour. It also enabled a shift in herself from good girl to powerful woman—a great psychological foundation for herself as emerging mother.

Endorphins

Endorphins can also trigger a crisis of confidence. This can seem counter-intuitive, because endorphins are often called the 'feel good' hormones. They are our natural opiates—surely they will make it all better? Well, yes and no, depending on your perspective. If your focus is on facilitating an efficient physiological labour and birth, then yes, they'll help. But if your perspective is about being pain free in labour, maybe not. Let me explain..

If the birthing woman has been supported to rise to the challenge of the building intensity without resorting to drugs or synthetic hormones that interfere with the normal physiological process then, at around 6–7 cm dilation in established first-stage labour, a further surge of hormones, including high levels of these endorphins, will flood her body.

Endorphins, as explained in chapter 3, increase the woman's birthing capacity in two ways. Firstly, by *moderating* her experience of pain, (yes moderating, *not* taking the pain away). And secondly (and to my mind more importantly), endorphins increase the woman's birthing capacity by swamping her cerebral cortex. This creates the 'shift in consciousness' (from thinking brain to primal brain) that unleashes the 'evolutionary regression' necessary for her instinctive birthing capacity to take over. When women surrender to this flood of endorphins the shift in consciousness brings both an inward-focused reverie—often appearing as if the birthing woman is falling asleep or is 'on the nod' as she rests between contractions—as well as enabling a primal instinctive release during the contractions.

Unfortunately this shift in consciousness, which is also an ego-dissolution process, far from being embraced for the birthing capacity it unlocks, is instead so often fearfully resisted. Instead of trusting it, many women experience this shift in consciousness as 'losing control'—losing control of their rational, civilised, ego-sense of being 'in control'.

'I observed that she was not used to losing control and was uncomfortable in her loss of control on every level,' remarked a colleague recently when reflecting on her support role in such a situation. It's a necessary surrender, similar to other creative processes, as Maria, from the physical theatre group Strange Fruit describes:

> It reminds me of the performing mind and the way that you have to surrender it, in terms of letting your ego go, to become almost a medium that channels something else to happen.[69]

To the inexperienced observer, the behaviours exhibited by a birthing woman surrendering and working with her birthing instincts and the behaviours of a birthing woman in the distress of a full-blown crisis of confidence, may both be confronting. However, there is a qualitative difference between a woman swept by hormonal surges into an evolutionary regression—who instinctively, rhythmically rocks, paces, sways, stamps, beats, moans, groans, wails, bellows, sings and roars—and a woman who, in a fearful, resistant, 'out of control' panic response, erratically thrashes about, with little awareness of her surroundings or situation.

Uninitiated birthing women themselves perhaps do not know, or trust that there is a difference. They may not have any body awareness that would enable them to trust the spontaneous movements and sounds that are expressions of their birthing instincts and so they may be more likely to resist the hormonally-driven shift in consciousness because they feel they are 'losing control' of themselves. These hormones and sensations can be experienced differently by each woman. One woman may be able to surrender instinctively, unrestrainedly, to her body's wisdom and so encounter a transcendent, transformative experience, while another woman may resist because she experiences herself as being unacceptably 'out of control'. Fearful of exposing her vulnerability, losing her rational control, or her sense of dignity, she tries to resist this necessary shift. Fuelled by this building resistance, a major crisis of confidence develops. Pain relief at this point, especially an epidural, seems to her like the only way to keep her dignity and limit any display of 'out of control' emotional vulnerability. She is culturally conditioned to think it's better to be a quiet, comfortable, passive, 'civilised' patient, than an active, instinctive, primal birthing woman.

Challenging labours

Some labours are more demanding than others, bringing up very challenging crises of confidence, usually because of the baby's position, an 'anterior lip', or a particularly long labour.

Anterior lip

An anterior lip occurs when most of the cervix is open. The baby's head is applying pressure on the remaining cervix or even slightly emerging from the uterus into the top of the vagina, causing a bearing-down urge to develop. Because the anterior or front of the cervix is still impeding the way, however, this causes a fiery crisis, as the mother tries to resist an irresistible bearing-down urge at the same time as the last of the cervix is being drawn up. Kaggi gives us a vivid description of an anterior lip crisis:

> The anterior lip of my cervix is not open and my midwife tells me I must not push. Is she mad? I feel the pushing urge in every cell of my body. But I trust her and with each contraction hold her hand and look into her eyes. We pant 'short short long' in rhythm together. She guides me and I follow as much as I can. It's so hard, my body is screaming with the urge to push.

Posterior labour

A posterior labour occurs when, instead of the baby's back being snugly spooned in the swell of the mother's belly, the curve of the baby's back is jammed up against the mother's lumbar curve. Kari's story gives us insight into the increased challenge of a long posterior labour:

> I had been in and out of pre- and early labour over forty hours. I had reached a point, physically, emotionally and mentally, where I needed some relief from the intensity, which had reached a new peak at that stage. My baby was bearing down on my back and I felt like I was going to explode into a million little pieces. I reached for the gas and it enabled me to stay with what was going on in my body, instead of trying desperately to will myself out. Although the gas took the edge off the searing intensity, I still found myself being pulled further and further into an abyss, and I was losing all control of my body. It no longer belonged to me—my baby was moving through and I was being remoulded with each contraction … I was wild-eyed with fear. I felt like I was being ripped open and I didn't know if I was going to survive, such was the level of my fear at that stage.

Kari did birth her baby, and as you'll see when we revisit her story in the next chapter, the experienced support she had in her facilitating holding circle enabled her to move through this fearful crisis.

Wild cards

For some women, the crisis of confidence may be more complexly layered with psychological issues. Internal patterning, or distressing life situations, events and traumas can act as unpredictable 'wild cards' in these women's labours. If you are a card player you will be familiar with wild cards. Or, if you follow tennis or other sports, or even politics for that matter, the idea of wild cards will also be familiar. In these contexts, a wild card represents a mixture of potency and unpredictability. You may not know when they are going to be played, you just know that when they are, they are guaranteed to have an impact.

We can apply this idea of wild cards to birthing. Particular life circumstances, issues and patterns can carry this unpredictable wild-card dynamic. We may not know when these life circumstances, issues or patterns will play out in the birth or postnatal period, or exactly what their effect will be. We just know that they will arise in some way.

Again, let me be clear. I'm not talking here about medical risk factors that require medically necessary interventions (although, if not adequately understood and supported, the flow-on effect of wild-card dynamics *can* be that medical interventions eventually become necessary). No, I'm referring to *psychosocial* risk factors, which can form part of the unconscious matrix. These are the invisible factors at work in birthing and mothering: emotions, fears, yearnings, relationships and personal history.

If understood, prepared for and supported, these wild card dynamics can bring forward opportunities for positive resolution and healing of old 'stuff'—psychological distress or trauma. On the other hand, if there is a lack of awareness or support, they can blindside birth intentions or hijack postnatal bliss.[70]

Sarah, whose early distress in labour first alerted me to the dynamics of a crisis of confidence and whose story I shared earlier, ended with this kind of healing magic. Late in her pregnancy, when the trust between us had deepened, she confided that she had a major wild card in her background. She revealed a distressing history of childhood sexual abuse and, given that she was a willing woman, she understood that in order to birth her baby without interventions, she would need to reclaim some deeply wounded places in her body and psyche. Recognising this, a large part of Sarah's late pregnancy preparations were spent in courageous, emotional work on this life wounding as it related to her birthing capacity. Later, in her birth story, she wrote:

> I had to shift an enormous amount of energy around the issue of feeling the world was safe for my baby girl. I had to grieve the lack of trust in which I lived.

During Sarah's labour, when I rushed to the birth centre, I experienced a mixture of feelings. Knowing the deep resistant energy which so often manifests in women with painful wild cards like Sarah's, I had predicted that this would be a long and difficult labour. Wild cards can create resistant energy causing an impasse, a blocked energy flow, which then affects the birth. It was this understanding that was informing my niggling intuition about Sarah's labour. As we heard earlier in this chapter, the midwife told me Sarah was already in 'transition'. My prediction of a long birth did not appear to be correct. I felt humbled. 'It's always good to have your pet theories exploded, Rhea', I thought to myself, although my intuitive niggle remained. I knew that the midwife was not aware of Sarah's background of sexual abuse, but it was my knowledge of this background that informed my unease. As you know from Sarah's story, after an early crisis of confidence her support team, informed by her commitment to the process, were able to support her to regroup and take the time needed for the demanding and painful process of holistic integration that would allow her to eventually birth her baby.

Sarah spent time 'howling into my cervix … the body's secrets, its memories, its terrors, its fears bared as labour broke the gates clouding the labyrinth of memory in my body', eventually not only birthing her baby, but also, as Sarah expressed it, giving herself 'the best chance of my deepest healing'.

Since Sarah's birthing I have been teaching about this 'crisis of confidence' concept and am happy that in the birth places that are proactive for normal physiological birth it has been recognised as a useful concept for birthing women, their support team and midwives. So, if you have heard the term already, before reading it in this book, and found it useful, then remember its genesis and be inspired by Sarah's determination and perseverance.

Undermining caregivers

Just as the quality of a caregiver's support and skills can sustain women through crises, birthing woman can also be catapulted into a crisis of confidence by undermining interactions with caregivers. 'It takes just one comment for it all to go to shit,' said Leigh, a mother of three, when discussing her first birth experience.

Sometimes undermining care occurs because of caregivers being stressed and overstretched; sometimes because of fear; sometimes because a caregiver is just having a 'bad day'; or sometimes because of the entrenched attitudes and birth-place power plays I've described earlier. Within the entrenched power hierarchies often found in our hospital systems the 'patients'—in this case the mothers and babies—sometimes find themselves on the bottom rung of the pecking order. And wherever there is an imbalance in power, controlling behaviours and victimisation can develop. There are big structural pressures at play here, which burden caregivers as well as mothers and babies. Whatever the cause, the effects on the mother of undermining care are usually the same—a crumbling into a self-belief crisis. Birth attendant Mandy describes such a scenario:

> She was about 4 cm dilated, handling her contractions very well. I'm sure it would have been helpful for her to know this, if the information had been presented to her in a positive way. Instead, her obstetrician said, 'I'm very disappointed in your progress; you are only 4 cm. I thought you would have done better than that by now', followed by a suggestion to use a drip to speed up her

> labour. She was crushed by his negative words and you could see her deflate. A crisis of confidence developed after this and didn't end till she was 10 cm and she started to push. So keeping her on track was a huge task for her support team.

Heather, another birth attendant, also describes this undermining care:

> By now she wanted an epidural as she was in so much pain. She looked to the midwife at this point and begged her with her voice and eyes to say something nice, something encouraging, to her to keep her going. The midwife just said, 'Something nice'. Not a help at all.

Sheryl's observations after the epidural-plus-forceps birth of her first baby illustrate some of the less-than-positive interactions with her stranger caregivers:

> Their condescending and patronising attitudes drove me crazy … every time they called me 'good girl' I felt like I was going to explode. It seemed like they kept sending messages about my incompetence. I fought it but as I got desperate I felt more and more dependent, like some sort of 'little girl' helplessness. Anyway, eventually I gave up and just did what they wanted.

All of the pathways to a crisis of confidence described above—physiological demand, hormones, emotional and psychological processes, undermining caregivers, challenging labours and wild cards—can, of course, act synergistically, creating multi-layered resistances in the birthing woman. These multi-layered crises can still be worked through, but they generally require caregivers who are experienced in the art of 'psychological interventions'. Even so, sometimes these crises of confidence can escalate to such levels of painful resistance that medical pain-relief options become appropriate. And sometimes these crises of confidence moments can, without facilitating support and guidance, develop into a medical crisis.

Crisis of confidence: consequences

The main consequence of an unsupported crisis of confidence is that it's often the start of the cascade of interventions. This cascade so often results from the way birthing women are 'nudged' at these vulnerable crisis moments, when they are highly susceptible to the influence of those around them. I see three pathways to this cascade of interventions. Firstly, the introduction of drugs, particularly epidurals, to manage a crisis of confidence can set off the cascade. Secondly, as we've seen earlier in the chapter, if the crisis of confidence response is misinterpreted as transition, then the deflation effect of this misinterpretation can also set off the cascade of interventions. Finally, an extended and unsupported emotional crisis of confidence may eventually result in problematic high levels of stress hormones in the mother and baby, which can create stalling or other medical crises, requiring interventions.

Pain-relief options used to manage any crisis of confidence are often the cause of further medical interventions. For instance, there is the case where the baby needs to be delivered by forceps or vacuum extraction and episiotomy because the mother is unable to effectively push after the effects of the epidural set up to manage her crisis of confidence. Then there's the baby who needs eventually to be delivered by an emergency caesarian, because its heart rate has plummeted in response to the epidural and drip combination used to speed up the labour as a solution to an earlier crisis of confidence brought on by misreading the crisis as transition.

As I've discussed in chapter 2, while there are some births that require interventions for true medical need, there are many labours that end in such 'unintended' medical interventions because they have been set off in the first place through labour-bypass era philosophies and protocols—and in particular because birthing women do not receive the intense support and guidance needed for working through any crises of confidence.

In my work as a counsellor working with birth issues, I hear many stories that illustrate the consequences of the failure to support women through these crises. For the willing woman, at the very least, such situations mean she experiences a diminished sense of herself with an eroded trust in her body and pain-threshold capacity. In more complex crises of confidence, underpinned by synergistic factors including wild cards and psychological distress, there is also the possibility that the results of these unsupported births and subsequent interventions can leave some women experiencing trauma reactions, post-natal depression or even post-traumatic stress disorder after the birth. This was the case for Wendy.

> It was more painful than I could ever have imagined and I had thought beforehand that if I got to a point in labour when I couldn't cope anymore then someone would guide me by helping me change positions or getting me into a hot shower or talking me through it—that's why I went to hospital. But despite asking for help it did not come and so I felt helpless with no control.

Due to her resulting adrenalised state, Wendy's labour then stalled, setting off the cascade of interventions.

> I found giving birth so horrible and seemed to relive the horror all the time and couldn't think about it without crying for at least a year. In hindsight I think I probably experienced some sort of PTSD. I certainly felt traumatised and suffered a physical and emotional crisis for some months.

I need to say here in response to the distress we hear in Wendy's story, that while I am, in the main, linking the research about known experienced caregivers with increasing potential for normal physiological birth, the continuity offered also leads to better emotional outcomes for birthing women after complex and difficult births.

Women can, of course, experience trauma responses during situations of medical crisis where interventions for true medical need are required. But trauma can also be experienced in situations where women experience unintended interventions after unsupported crises of confidence have hijacked their labours[71]. Erin said, after the birth of her first child:

> I had great difficulty understanding and processing her birth, I suffered from nightmares, flashbacks, anxiety, anger and sadness. I was in conflict because, on paper, it looked like a healthy birth—so it was difficult to get help. Friends assumed that, because I didn't have a c-section, I had a good natural birth, but to me it was far from natural. I felt silenced by those who gave me the line about 'a healthy baby being all that mattered'.[72]

Surely we should be trying to avoid as many of these unnecessary trauma reactions as we can.

Crisis of confidence: working through

The ability to work physically with a crisis of confidence needs first to be underpinned by some key understandings. I've already mentioned these but they bear repeating: normalising functional, physiological pain and separating that from issues of medical danger; having a 'growth' mindset that sees benefit in undertaking experiences that extend us beyond our existing limits; and, finally, knowing you don't have to *like* every moment of the labour in order to do it well. Remember the willing woman's mantra—*I don't need to like it to do it brilliantly!* Then, the willing woman who yearns for the peak experience of normal physiological birthing, is best served if she can normalise and also plan for this experience of a crisis of confidence. For some women, their previous lived experiences have developed in them mental, emotional, physical and spiritual resources that they can draw on when a crisis erupts. This was the case for Jill.

> I was only 2 cm dilated—after all that time we hadn't even really begun. I became so disillusioned. I had a hot shower. It was here that my emotions were unleashed—I was overcome by tears and disappointment, feeling like such a failure that at such an early stage I felt like I needed pain relief! What was happening? What

> happened to all my ideals? How full of shit I was! All great in theory, but when it came to the reality I couldn't carry it out—an intense sense of failure. After a few tears, and many kind and reassuring words later, I spent a few moments in the shower on my own and asked my goddess to please show me the way through; to show me the way to work with her; to surrender and let it happen. And indeed it did! From that moment on something changed, something shifted.

There are also women whose habitual body engagement has fully supported them to match the demands and challenges of birthing. Their self-regulated responses enable them to move through any momentary disorganisation, thus averting the development of a full-blown crisis. Natalie, a dancer, dance instructor and dance therapist, illustrates this capacity beautifully in describing her first birth experience:

> At some point I felt a real wave and change-up a gear in terms of the surges. I felt a little shocked at the change and the power of the surge. For the slightest moment I thought, 'My God, it's going to keep on coming and I am not going to be able to handle this'. But the next few big waves came and I concentrated and then they became the norm. I added my voice to the out breath, like a humming or 'ahhhhh' sound. I directed my breath and voice to a point just in front of me and kind of outwards and sometimes downwards. The surges intensified and I really had to use my voice and push into the furniture to feel safe enough to cope with the pain. I felt another few changes up in gear and one in particular caught me by surprise. I had to tell myself not to panic. I realised I had been thinking that I was in fifth gear before but that now I was in fifth! Soon that intensity also became the norm. And later still … another surge and out slides the baby in a gush of warm fluid. Glendyn passes the baby through my legs and I hold him in my hands and look … I can't believe it is a baby. It is a little boy. I hold the little warm and wet baby up to my breast and give him a hug.

Even if you haven't previously engaged with physical exertion to any great degree, however, you can still prepare yourself for the physical demands of labour. Willing women whose life experiences have not previously developed appropriate body knowledge and internal resources would best use their pre-pregnancy and pregnancy as a time to undertake focused regular practise: increasing their fitness, stamina and 'working with pain' capacity, perhaps through walking, swimming, pregnancy yoga, physio, stretch or dance classes. They could also practise breathing, relaxation and body-awareness release processes—in order to develop this capacity and resilience.

All this body preparation will help when it comes to a crisis of confidence, but there are also willing women who, because of wise choices, find themselves in optimal birthing contexts (including the ambience in the birth space), and so find their susceptibility to a crisis of confidence minimised. I know I've said earlier that you will have a crisis of confidence, *but* in well-supported situations some birthing women who are on that edge of a possible crisis will, like Penny, be able to shift gears and accommodate the building intensity without a fully blown crisis unfolding.

> The happiest moment was when we heard that I was ready to push. I hadn't reached the end of my tether, I hadn't started begging for pain-relief medication (it hadn't even occurred to me), and I was reasonably awake and alert.

Normalising a crisis of confidence

It's my hope that my 'normalising' crisis of confidence moments by placing labour on a spectrum of peak-performance and challenging life experiences (whether physical, creative, academic or spiritual), will support willing women. Not by rescuing them from these crises, but rather by encouraging realistic awareness, so that a willing woman struggling with such a crisis might herself be reassured. Irma attended my 'Embracing the Intensity' workshop, in which I describe this crisis:

> Understanding what a crisis of confidence was before I went into labour helped both my husband and me enormously. Nine hours into the labour the midwife did an internal exam and reported that I was only 2 cm dilated. I couldn't believe it. After all those hours of hard work I thought I must have been at least 6 cm (although I was secretly hoping to discover that I was closer to ten!). 'Don't worry' she said to me, trying to be reassuring. 'It'll probably only take another five or six hours to get there.' Well, by this point I was already so exhausted that the thought of another five hours seemed absolutely impossible. I broke down in tears, my face pressed into the bed, feeling utterly hopeless. And yet despite this, despite the fact that I was moaning 'I just can't do it', a part of me was also calmly and rationally thinking, 'Ah! So this is a crisis of confidence'. This knowledge reassured me, it normalised the experience and actually robbed the crisis of the power it might have had. I knew that it was an expected part of the labour process and that, like all those women before me, I would get through it. This knowledge helped my husband, too, who was calmly stroking my back and reassuring me that I could do it. In the end my crisis lasted only a minute or two and by the time the next contraction hit I was ready to go, and in fact went on to make it through another fifteen hours (with another crisis when I realised I had been labouring through a night, a day and was into night again!) before greeting my baby girl.

A savvy, willing birthing woman will have made wise choices in support of her capacity and therefore surrounded herself with experienced support people who are able to celebrate her potency and encourage her to extend herself into the unfamiliar, uncomfortable, painful demands of her labour. This is the support needed for moving through any crisis of confidence, and it will increase her resilience and sense of achievement, as Irma confirms as she continues her reflection on the normal physiological birth of her daughter:

> Looking back on the labour of my first child I felt an overwhelming sense of pride. I had made it through twenty-four hours of painful posterior labour without drugs or intervention to bring my baby into the world. Honestly, you could have handed me the Booker Prize or Olympic gold and it would have meant nothing in comparison. The sense of achievement was incomparable.

Surely this inspirational experience would serve Irma, or any other birthing woman, as a solid self-affirming foundation for her journey on into mothering?

Conclusion

Making a distinction between transition and what I am calling a crisis of confidence is important for the willing woman. Reframing and normalising crisis of confidence moments is also important for willing women. And understanding that when a crisis of confidence is on, with emotional distress running high and the willing woman herself feels she cannot find a way through, support can make the difference. The remedy for a crisis of confidence is support that can get you through. This is what we are going to explore in greater depth in the next chapter.

Personal reflection

- Have you had experiences that have developed your capacity to work through pain-tolerance levels?
- Have you experienced crisis of confidence moments in any area of your life?
- Do you have a patterned response to crisis of confidence experiences?
- Do you have any awareness of how your patterned response developed?
- How do these patterns play out in your self-talk and behaviours?
- What personal or family pain response patterns might surface in labour?
- What might the implications be for your birthing?
- Who will support you through any crisis of confidence?
- What do you need to set in place for your best possibility of working through any crisis of confidence in labour?
- Have you felt the unburdening and satisfaction of cathartic release?
- Are there any wild-card issues you'll need to be aware of?
- Do you have experienced support for any 'wild cards' that may arise?
- Do you feel any emotional or psychological resistance to releasing your baby into your world?

6

The right support: who will get you through?

Waves of confidence coming at her—that's the antidote to a birthing woman's crisis of confidence.

'I was hit by this powerful sound,' says Kristy, recalling the time when, as a teenager, she had arrived at the homebirth of one of her new cousins. 'It made me anxious but I looked at the midwives. They were all quiet and relaxed, so I took my cue from them.'

Later in her life, when she went on to have her own children, Kristy felt again the waves of confidence offered by this supportive calmness in her own facilitating holding circle.

> Birthing my daughter at home surrounded by people I knew and trusted, I found to be the most powerful and transformative experience I have ever had. I went to the depths of my primal soul and found strength that I never knew I had. Being surrounded by people who believed in me and trusted the birth process, who

> knew what to do to support a woman in labour was essential. I had a strong belief in myself and that my body could do it, but their reassuring words and encouraging faces dispelled even any fleeting doubts.
>
> The birth of my first daughter left me feeling strong, empowered and confident. Those few short hours of birthing my child taught me a lot about my inner strength and power. Since then I have talked to a lot of other mothers and it is very rare to hear other stories of empowerment. The prevailing stories are of 'bad' birth experiences, intervention and disempowerment. Women are missing out on this valuable experience. This is why I want to be a birth attendant and eventually a midwife. Because it is the support of the people around you that can make the crucial difference in what type of birth experience you have. If they have confidence in you and the birthing process, it's easier to have confidence in yourself.

Remember my description in chapter 4 of the 'circles of influence' surrounding birthing women? Well, now we're hitting the two inner circles in that description—the 'circle of birth-place culture' and the 'circle of known support'. Has the willing woman made wise choices to set up a facilitating environment for the work of labour—a *facilitating holding circle*? Or has she chosen a *naïve support circle*, who will want to save her from any distress?

It is all going to be revealed when everybody's resolve is put to the test during a crisis of confidence. What's coming at the birthing woman then—waves of confidence? Or waves of sympathy and fear?

Facilitating environment for achievement

In the world of intense physical engagement undertaken as a pathway towards personal-best or peak performance, we understand the vital role that support plays.

In fact, in the conversations I'm sharing with you, everybody acknowledged what marathon swimmer Tammy van Wisse emphasised when she said, during our interview:[73]

> The quality of support can make the difference between achieving something mediocre and something great.

Tammy described the balance required between an individual's capacity on the one hand, and the support needed to maximise that capacity on the other. She explains:

> If you try and draw on your own inner strength and that's not working, you might come back and say 'Hey I'm struggling here, help me'. You need to use your support team's energy and rely on them to get through that particular point of time. We all try and be strong and self-reliant and think 'I can do this on my own', but in truth we all need the support of people. The more you can open up to that aspect and rely on people to help you through, then the better the outcome will be.

Can you imagine Tammy, inside her shark cage, making her seventeen-hour Bass Strait swim without a circle of supporters who believed in her and knew how to urge her on as she was hitting hard against pain and stamina barriers—hitting crises of confidence? To get through these crises, she needed supporters able to buoy her with their waves of confidence.

> I was crying, the guys from the Royal Life Saving Society—it was night time and they were jumping into the shark cage. It was freezing and they didn't have wetsuits on and they were standing at the side of the cage holding a spotlight, holding a torch and saying 'Stay with me, stay with me, I believe in you, stay with me', and they were swapping, they were taking turns, fifteen minutes each, and I was swimming, just trying to look at the light on the bottom of the cage and just stay with them.

I think back to the memories I have of encouraging students into new challenging physical experiences—deep water and survival swimming, working on high rope courses, abseiling, rock climbing. Now I acknowledge that, of course, there were safety needs and a skill-set to be taught: how to move the arms for that particular stroke, how to adjust the ropes and harnesses, how to find the next hand and foot hold. But the most important aspect of that teaching role was to provide a psychologically supportive environment, a 'facilitating environment' that was able to protect the student from any self-doubts and contain the fear and anxiety of a crisis of confidence—while simultaneously encouraging them towards the achievement and enjoyment of a new activity.

Maria, from the physical performance ensemble Strange Fruit, spoke to me[74] about this need for a facilitating environment to encourage her through self-doubts, when she described her first experience of getting on the performance apparatus—6 m-high flexible fibreglass 'sway poles', which the performers are strapped into, before sweeping and swaying in awe-inspiring rhythm and movement.

> That did bring up psychological roots about learning and self-image. My judgemental thinking put me down mentally and that would cause tensions in my body and make it harder. So it can become a vicious circle, because when I hit a wall in my mind, then my body becomes less capable of doing it or relaxing and surrendering into it.
>
> Then the kind of support I get either helps or doesn't. The support could trigger my own judgemental voice. I always have to work with these self-doubts anyway, so if there's someone even slightly pushing that button as well ... You want to access a power of vulnerability in creative work as well as in birth, so you need a non-judgemental safe environment, you need that holding circle to give you that space.

I'm often asked by people who know my work whether I've seen this or that 'crisis of confidence' unfold on last night's reality TV show?

I'm told that crises of confidence are erupting all over the place on these shows—dancers and singers; chefs and survivors; weight loss, make-over and quiz contestants, all experiencing the crumbling distress of a crisis of confidence. And just as it is in births, the quality of support here is crucial. It seems there's plenty of support flowing to the contestants, willing them on, wanting them to move past their limitations to achieve their goals. Maybe I should start watching?

Performer Nancy Sposato[75] told me she saw a parallel between her performance work and birthing. She felt that for the birth of her son, and in her performance, she required others, a 'support team' to affirm her, listen to her and get her through:

> It was support that helped me overcome the 'emotional blocks' that arise when you are revealing the vulnerability that you feel, the bringing of your authenticity to the surface. I had a support team for my piece *A Room Within* and a support team for my birth as well; it was a love-fest.

Playwright and novelist Joanna Murray-Smith spoke to me[76] about the painful confrontation with self and the support needed to enable the fullest expression of her creative energy:

> I know that the only good writing that will come out of an idea will be writing that is mined from a very deep place and I know that is going to be difficult, going to be painful and I know from the outset it's going to involve a surrendering. And if you've got enough good people around you, then that's where you get the courage to surrender to the journey.

Playwright, writer and dramaturge Andrew Bovell reinforced the point during our interview[77] when he elaborated on this issue of painful creative process with actors and the need for a supportive facilitating environment:

> A lot of the workshop or rehearsal processes are about creating an environment in which risks can be taken safely. The risk might be looking stupid, revealing parts of your body, revealing parts of your emotional psyche, making bold gestures in your performance. When there's the trust in the rehearsal room an actor will keep working, keep taking risks. Good actors will keep working with difficult material. Geoffrey Rush was a good example on the film *Lantana*. We'd be in rehearsal and he'd be struggling and struggling … then finally he'd say it a different way and it was exactly right.
>
> And that certainly applies in the writing process as well—creating the circumstance in which you feel that you can take risks, because out of those risks the surprising or unexpected things come. But you know, good directors, good managers of the process know how to do that safely, like good midwives do.

You can see here that I'm again expanding my idea of a crisis of confidence to cover the whole gamut of challenging human endeavours and drawing out the understanding that when we are struggling and feel we can't go on, our achievement is often dependant on the quality of support we receive. This is the function of a facilitating environment.

I was reminded of all this recently when a friend sent a text after completing a parachute jump: 'Oh my god! Just did the jump. Scariest thing ever! But fantastic!' I'm pretty sure jump instructors must know a thing or two about creating a facilitating environment.

I was also reminded of this need for a facilitating environment to continue working through potential crisis moments of effort, endurance and self-belief when I was out on my walk this morning. Straining up a killer rise, I was overtaken by an equally straining small group of jogging, stroller-pushing new mums. I was struggling near the top, and the mums were too (if I was reading their ragged breathing and facial grimacing correctly). They appeared in danger of succumbing to the familiar flagging resolve brought on by an 'I can't do it' voice in their heads. Their personal trainer, with exquisite timing, in an encouraging yet determined tone, provided the 'facilitating' motivation: 'That's it, you're all doing great, keep breathing into those legs, keep that rhythm going'.

Immediately the cacophony of struggling, gasping breaths shifted into a rhythmic focused unison as they pushed on to the top. As they moved away from me, I watched them with their new babies, and hoped that they had 'backed' their birthing potential with such facilitating expertise in the same way as they were 'backing' their fitness and wellbeing now.

Core concepts of support

What have you not accomplished in your life because you haven't felt safe enough? What have you missed out on because you haven't been encouraged or supported through the distress of confronting your vulnerability, fear of failure or whatever your particular brand of personal sabotage might be?

How many challenging, anxiety-making, yet personally expansive, exhilarating or strengthening activities have you either done or not done, because of the support—the *holding*—you did or did not receive?

When we contemplate these questions we are taken into the psychological realm of accomplishment and the psychological dynamics of support for achievement.

'Holding'

The idea of 'holding' that I'm using here when I talk about the facilitating holding circle, was developed as a theoretical concept by paediatrician and psychotherapist DW Winnicott.[78]

He explained that psychology is a gradual extension of physiology; that the way a baby is physically held will be transcribed into the child's psychological development. And that the act of holding can be understood to also represent a metaphorical holding.

Like Winnicott, I am extending the idea of holding at a birth from actual physical holding, to include the more psychological, energetic and symbolic forms of holding that Winnicott called a 'facilitating environment', and which I am also using to describe the function of the facilitating holding circle.

Now, to come to my idea of the facilitating holding circle, I'm drawing on my awareness of birth process, birth culture, birth support and pain dynamics, as well as psychological theories. Finally, I'm drawing on an understanding of the support needs of anyone engaged in striving for achievement.

It's easier to grasp this use of 'holding' as an energetic concept if we start from something physical. Beth Shelton, dancer and choreographer, spoke to me[79] about dancers creating a facilitating holding environment for each other:

> It all becomes a network of energy rather than simply one body struggling away on its own. It's immensely supportive in terms of getting past a 'can't keep your breath' barrier, a stamina barrier, a pain barrier. It gives you that sense of holding, of something facilitating, something wider than your own body that kind of participates … and supports you.

Actor Eugenia Fragos also spoke to me[80] about the feeling of being 'held' in her creative process:

> A good director will be on to it before I am. Some directors will see the germ of where I'm stuck and struggling and will create the opportunity to move through it. And so you have an experience of that circle of holding, the safety net—that they are 'being with you'.

Andrew Bovell, too, spoke about this facilitative energetic holding when he described the facilitating holding circle that sustains his work:

> … an understanding partner, a physical space and a mental space. Then the other parts of my holding circle are five or six people whom I trust and who believe in me and my writing.

Holding can also be recognised as a spiritual or religious concept. Sending positive thoughts to another, holding them in your thoughts, saying prayers for another, surrounding someone in white light or lighting a candle for them—these are all examples of energetic holding.

Empathy versus sympathy

In my workshops and presentations I flash two images on the screen. The first is of 400 m Olympic gold medallist Cathy Freeman. Functional pain is written all over her face—grimacing, striving to the limit, straining for achievement. And what is our response to such an image? We can see she's in pain but do we pity her, feel sympathy for her? No, our response is *Go Cathy!* We celebrate her effort and revel in her achievement, pain and all.

I then show an image of a birthing woman in a birth tub, working with her body—functional pain written all over her face, grimacing, striving to the limit. This always creates an 'ah-ha' moment, as everyone in the room 'gets it'. They all see how we are so programmed to pity birthing women, to see them as suffering rather than seeing their achievement. Willing women and their support teams have some serious reframing to do!

Empathy? Yes, of course, there's plenty of empathy required in the facilitating holding circle. What psychiatrist Heinz Kohut calls 'the accepting, confirming and understanding human echo'.[81] Yes, we need plenty of that 'psychological nutrient' to supplement the birthing woman's resolve. But *no sympathy!*

'No sympathy' was a core concept articulated by everyone I spoke to about facilitating achievement. They all spoke equally strongly on this issue of the absolute need to eliminate sympathy and pity from the 'network of energy' surrounding them.

Anglican priest Anna spoke clearly on this issue of 'no sympathy' when I interviewed her[82] about her work as a spiritual counsellor:

> Some people just go over and over the same ground and want me to be sympathetic or to do the work for them. I have to encourage them. I can't do the work for them and I'm not really interested

> in being sympathetic. I will help them but they will be doing the work and I will be encouraging them. Sympathy and pity are very debilitating and definitely not on the agenda.

I asked Tammy van Wisse what would have happened at a crisis time if her support crew, instead of encouraging her on, had become fearful and began offering her sympathy? *'I wouldn't make it,'* was her emphatic reply!

> My Mum and Dad never come on the support boat because my Mum says that if she saw me 'suffering' she'd have me pulled out of the water in about two minutes. She can't stand to see me in pain, so I know she'd be useless.

Before her Bass Strait swim, Tammy needed to make clear support choices to back her intentions:

> It's very much an organisational skill, in that you have to really know the people you have involved. You do need to say to them, 'If I get really emotional, because I'm in so much pain, please don't sympathise with me because I really want to do this. I want to get through this and I want you to help me, even if I'm crying out. So can you do that?' And if they say, 'No, I couldn't see you in pain', then you know that that's not the person for you. You really do need to refine it. I did a lot of research, till I was comfortable, and could say, 'Right, that's the person for me; I know they can do their job'.

And what is their job at a birth? Well, one part of their job is to be able to witness painful effort without succumbing to their own distress.

If there is sympathy and pity in the birth space this will generally mean that members of the support team are also suffering and in distress. So sometimes pain-relief options are just as appealing (or more so!) to the support team as they are to the birthing woman herself. Not that the support team are taking the drugs, but when the birthing woman accesses the drugs or the epidural it has the 'bonus' effect of settling the emotional discomfort experienced by partners or others in the birth team who are distressed by witnessing the birthing woman in pain. In fact, a need to take care of their support team is sometimes a trigger for women choosing pain relief in the first place.

Father and comedian Adam Vincent, on his 'Dad's blog'[83], refers to this sympathy-suffering dynamic:

> Witnessing pain is hard. Yes, it's not as tough as experiencing the pain of childbirth. No, men will never get to wear that badge of honour. But really there is a 'watching someone go through pain' threshold. And as a man you have to push through that 'witnessing pain' pain barrier. You'll beg for drugs but you'll be denied. Some rubbish about hospital policy!

Experienced support

There are crucial moments, crisis of confidence moments, where a birthing woman's sense of a way forward needs to be supported by waves of confidence offered by women who have walked through this wilderness before. The need for support experienced in the skills of working with pain and endurance, is needed.

If a birthing woman doesn't have experienced support women with her then her male partner will lovingly, diligently, try to 'go there' with her—but then you're likely to face what I call the 'what the fuck would you know?' moment!

This 'what the fuck would you know?' response to her partner's reassuring words at these crucial moments—often spoken, sometimes unspoken (but eloquently communicated by the birthing woman through a flash of eyes and body language)—speaks to a lack of credibility. He may mean well and be saying all the right things, but he just doesn't have the credibility to hold it together, the credibility of someone who has been there before.

This can often become the point of crumbling of the birthing woman's resolve, with consequences for the fulfilment of her aspirations for a normal physiological birth—especially if the partner is her main or sole support.

Susan Maushart, author and social commentator, in a presentation at a homebirth conference in Canberra, alluded to this dynamic.

> Why, at the moment in our lives when we will most need expert nurturing, do we choose to put ourselves in the hands of amateurs?

Maria from Strange Fruit emphasises the importance of 'that trust that a person knows what they are talking about. It's a lot harder working with a director who hasn't got the physical experience of the apparatus, as opposed to someone who has done a lot of performances'.

Of course, that's not only true in physical performance, as theatre director Jenny Kemp explained in our interview:[84]

> I mean one has to actually encourage relationship with that difficult stuff, that hard stuff, that stuff that actors often feel is bad. You don't just get it from an actor. Because I've noticed with actors when we're rehearsing and the actor is being what I call really wonderful and courageous, and spontaneous, daring to be what feels to them as if they're out of control, when in fact it isn't. But it feels unrecognisable and scary to them. Now that's a very vulnerable moment. And I say 'that was really wonderful, give me more of that'.

This is again like birth. The birthing woman on that ego-dissolving evolutionary regression, making sounds and moving instinctively, directed by the strong contractions throwing her about—she comes off the contraction feeling 'Oh, I don't like this, I'm losing control, I'm not coping well'. And the experienced support person says 'That's fantastic, it's going well, we want more of that'.

I remember again, in my conversation with Tammy van Wisse, her describing a situation in which Dawn Fraser, her mentor, had the credibility factor covered, and so offered experienced, strengthening energy at a demanding crisis in Tammy's seventeen-hour Bass Strait swim.

> I can't stand it anymore and I'm crying and I want to get out, and that's when a lot of my support people turn away, they can't see me like that and I don't need to see them being upset and crying. Dawn will be the strong one and say, 'Well, how much do you want it? How much do you want it, you've come this far, you are so close, do you really want to give up now?' And I think to myself 'No, I don't, I don't. I'm in a lot of pain but I've come this far and I'd be stupid to give it all away now. This is what I wanted to do, I put myself in this situation, I've trained for it, I've planned for it, I want to do it!'
>
> I guess you've got to be hungry for it, but then again, you've got to have somebody who can put your focus back into that. So you really do need that person who's going to really know what to do and be your strength when you need it. So that's why Dawn is such an inspiration, she gets me through the really bad times.

Many births, particularly first births, require the mother to complete her own form of marathon—mentally, emotionally and physically. Who will be her inspiration, her mentor, her 'Dawn Fraser'? Who will get her through the really bad times?

You will remember Kari's posterior birth marathon from the last chapter. Luckily, she had her own experienced support, her own 'Dawn Fraser', to see her through the really bad times in her labour.

> She had come in and sat quietly and lovingly beside me—really taking in where I was at that point. And I felt myself sigh with relief at the level of support just her presence had brought to me. She was solid and grounded, and sat with me through the roller coaster ride of each contraction. She sensed me then, moving further into a wild place, and she stepped more fully into my awareness than she had been.
>
> She encouraged me to keep my eyes open, which I found so challenging, but it enabled me to keep a hold on my actual reality of being in that tub, being in that room. She held my gaze, she touched my head and she was absolutely right there with me every

> step of the way. Each tidal wave of contraction that hit me, she held me with her eyes, her voice, and her strength. I was a wild animal, frenzied, looking into the eyes of a deeply centred being, emanating wisdom and safety. In that safety, the fear had no place and began to melt. And so I hung onto her in this way until I just allowed my body to let go and allowed the forces of creation to fully open me for birth.

It seemed to me during these conversations about support that the feeling and skill of a good 'Dawn Fraser', or a facilitating director, who enables an actor to feel safe enough to trust, be in touch with and then to surrender to their own creative expression, parallels so closely the profound skill of a facilitating midwife or an experienced birth attendant. The skill of a facilitating support person in birth is to enable the birthing woman to feel safe so she can trust the birth process and her body enough to surrender to the experience of intense birthing energy flowing through her. Independent midwife Jennie Teskey explains what's required:

> Just total love and trust and believing in the process … believing in her ability. And that you are at ease with whatever may come up, like the regression, the torment, the struggle. That you are prepared to journey it with them, to not waver and not feel too tired and want to give up yourself. It's having that strength and trust.

Protect against self-doubt

Not all of us have personal difficulties with self-doubts. However, the abundance of advice and information on how to change our negative thinking and self-talk would suggest that many of us do. Coupled with these general patterns of self-doubt, contemporary birthing women cannot help but be sensitised by the pervasive negativity and fear regarding birth that bombards them from the wider culture.

So, ideally, willing women will surround themselves with a facilitating holding circle able to protect them from their own self-doubts, to hold their disintegrating self-belief together, as well as 'quelling the acculturated inner voice' of doubting messages living in their psyche—as birthing mother Tamara described it.

The function of the facilitating holding circle is not to 'save' the willing woman from the effort-filled and often painful work of birthing, but rather to save her from her own perceived limitations—her self-doubts, fears, resistances and any inhibiting life patterns that may undermine her physical stamina and emotional resourcefulness.

The facilitating holding circle holds a trust that normal physiological childbirth is achievable. Those in this circle hold a trust that this woman is resourceful and resilient enough to work with her labour, as they also encourage her towards its building intensity.

The function of the holding circle is to hold all this trust in a solid, grounded, energetic 'containing', which is felt by the birthing woman as a solid circle of support that can be leaned into and drawn on to bolster her own flagging energy, intention or trust. When there is commitment and expertise in the facilitating holding circle a potent energetic container emerges that offers the mother an unassailable circle of support.

Remember Sally's exhilarating story from the previous chapter? After backing her intention of normal physiological birth with focused preparation, she then, during the labour, continued on through a number of crises, to eventually birth her beautiful daughter in exactly the way she had desired. Such a demanding birth does not usually unfold in this way without a potent holding circle.

Tess's story

I'm also reminded of another story where the birthing woman's awareness of the strength and resolve in her holding circle left no oxygen to fan her fears. After the home water birth of her bonny boy—as she luxuriated with him and we all enjoyed cake and champagne—Tess's sister (who had previously had two homebirths) was enthusiastically congratulating her. 'You were fantastic and you didn't even have a crisis of confidence,' her sister said.

Tess, the new mother, laughed and revealed that she had, in fact, struggled with many crises across the labour, during which she had resolved to herself that for her next birth she would not get trapped at home again with no escape to an epidural! She said that there were times when she wanted to grab the car keys and drive herself to hospital to get that epidural. Then she would look around her support circle and see everyone's shining faces and hear our encouraging words and she felt that there was no use in even voicing her doubts; no use in even whimpering or whinging; no use wasting any energy complaining. There was nothing else for it but to get on with it and let our belief in her and in birth, carry her through.

This feeling of being trapped, like Tess, usually marks the bottom of a distress spiral. Then, supported by waves of confidence, the birthing woman is held through her crisis and buoyed long enough to catch a new wave of confidence and ride it to the shore. So there's a story of a successful facilitating environment, a facilitating holding circle able to contain Tess's distress, holding her to her intentions and capacity for birthing. And two years later, surrounded by the same facilitating holding circle she birthed her second baby at home in that same birth tub!

Accepting functional pain

You can see that another core concept in the facilitating holding circle needs to be an acceptance and normalising of functional, physiological pain.

Caregivers and support people of a willing woman must be able to normalise the pain of labour, believe in her body's hormonal capacity to respond to the intensity and believe in her ability to work with it.

You can hear this sense of normalising the pain and effort in these comments from Jan, an experienced midwife:

> If others with the woman are disturbed by the yells of the labouring woman, the midwife just continues doing what she's doing, she's not shocked.

The entire support team must be shaped around an acceptance of and an ability to work with the reality of the healthy functional pain that is inevitably part of the territory of peak-performance activities. This understanding and skill within the support team will enable the members of the circle to hold steadfast to the intentions of the willing woman they are supporting and enable them to bring her back to her focus at those times when she herself is struggling to maintain her own energy and belief.

Sonia also gives us some insight into the different types of support required to get through a tough challenge when she talks about her experience of completing the 100 km Oxfam Trailwalker Challenge over thirty-six hours.

> Different stages of the walk required different types of support. In the early stages it was all about the practical stuff. The team's energy was high and the adrenalin and excitement were getting us through. Of course, the training played a huge part, too, but as the night set in the adrenalin was gone and we were further than we'd ever walked in training; then the support crew became so much more important. A hot dinner at the checkpoint, wrapping me in blankets, making me hydrate and eat plenty of food without me needing to ask for anything.
>
> All that practical support was essential, there's no way we could do it without that. But when my Mum was clocking off support duties and our night crew was taking over I got really shaky and sad—I felt like a little kid and it was my first glimpse of how much emotional support and holding I had been getting from her as well.
>
> The worst bit for me was at about one-thirty in the morning, we were about 60 km in and we had been walking since seven in the morning. We thought we would be at the sleep checkpoint by this time and we'd been told there weren't any more hills in this section of the trail, but there were tonnes of them, so the whole team was starting to lose it and yell at the ground and curse

the whole thing. Going up these hills was just awful. About that time I got a text message from Dad asking how it was going and I responded with a big whinge about how I was tired and how it felt like we were all falling apart. I was really looking for sympathy at that point but instead Dad just accepted where I was at and with complete calm he wrote, 'Ah, a clear night, a canopy of stars and good friends for companions. All is well.' Everything within me went calm, and I was okay to push through to the next stop. Just knowing that someone was awake with me in the night when I was feeling so alone, believing I could do it; that got me through.

Giving your support team the green light

Underlying the dynamics within the holding circle are two other linked issues. One is what I call the 'green light' issue. I've mentioned it before, with regard to identifying yourself and your intentions to the midwife. But it's also necessary to give your support team a green light.

Before the labour, a willing woman needs to give her facilitating holding circle a green light, giving them permission to support her through any crisis of confidence even when it looks pretty rugged. With a green light, specific support plans can be developed.

Medical practitioners Groopman and Hartzband in their book *Your Medical Choices: how to decide what is right for you*[85], mentioned earlier, report that 'George Lowenstein of Carnegie Mellon University, who has done extensive studies in decision-making, distinguishes between "hot" and "cold" emotional states.' They go on to say that Lowenstein explains, 'when we are in pain, anxious, angry, or frustrated, we are "hot" and prone to make choices that we imagine will quickly improve our condition'. A crisis of confidence is certainly a 'hot' state, which is why savvy willing women need to give a green light before the labour, when they are in a 'cold', more intentional state—in order to be able to be supported to resist the seduction of the epidural when they are in a 'hot' crisis state during the labour.

Thaler and Sunstein's 'nudge'[86] concept also adds weight to this 'green light' idea. In order to boost our capacity to resist temptation it's useful to understand that self-control issues arise when choices and their consequences are separated in time. Thaler and Sunstein talk about 'investment goods', where costs are born immediately but benefits are delayed. For instance, the effort of beginning an exercise program (early waking, aching muscles, etc) and the likelihood of crumbling motivation before improvements in fitness and wellbeing are experienced, or in our case, the effort of working with painful contractions right now and the time before the actual pay off of exhilaration and bonding promised by normal physiological birth. They also mention 'sinful goods', where we get the pleasure now but suffer the consequences later, you know, the sweet seduction of a packet of Tim Tams now and the remorse later. But more troubling in our case, we have the sweet seduction of the epidural now and the unintended consequences of the cascade of interventions later.

This idea of a green light then is really to increase your capacity to follow through on your savvy willing woman intentions, to use your support team to bridge any gap that may open up between your original intentions and the choices you may make in a 'hot' moment.

This is where a facilitating holding circle, given a green light and set up to support her birthing capacity, can make the greatest difference to a willing woman. In the midst of a crisis of confidence, which instincts are going to prevail—her birthing instincts, or her pain-avoiding instincts? Which instincts are going to be amplified by her holding circle? Will it be her 'Yes, I can' or her 'No, I can't'?

The other issue is the touchy matter in the heat of labour, of distracting, denying or refusing women when they are pleading for epidurals. As you can imagine, there's obviously an art to this, because it's not just about denying her the epidural she is fixated on. It's about having the expertise to offer *other* support measures to soothe and guide her.

This certainly needs discussion before the labour and will require everybody understanding that even though the birthing woman is demanding 'saving' in the distressing moment, the support team are holding to the bigger picture of her intentions.

If, however, all the 'working with pain' skills and creative options have been tried and still, over time, the birthing woman cannot be dissuaded from her fixation on an epidural, then the birth team may need to reconsider. Nonetheless, it can be tricky.

It bears repeating here that it's a different story if there are any 'true medical needs'—indications that the labour needs a different pathway. When I talk about the issue of dissuading a birthing woman from an epidural I'm speaking specifically about crises of confidence arising from the *normal, healthy, painful* effort of a normal physiological birth.

The siren song of the epidural

Willing women need to plan strategically to protect themselves from the seduction of the epidural that I've referred to in earlier chapters. My colleague Stef explained recently:

> Rose was crying for pain relief—she wanted out of the pain, not to feel the contractions anymore and she was being highly emotional, physically thrashing about, and screaming for the epidural. Her emotion was wild and she was refusing to let us access her.

When a willing woman like Rose has reached this fixation on an epidural, her support team really have their work cut out for them if they are going to honour her previous intention for normal physiological birth.

In my workshops, I've come to describe what I call the 'siren song' of the epidural. The seductive pull of this siren song is ubiquitous and entirely undermining of a birthing woman's resolve, confidence and resilience. So I suggest that if normal physiological birth is important to you then perhaps, like Ulysses, you need to have yourself 'strapped to the mast' in order to protect yourself from this siren song.

Experienced support can provide that mast, enabling safe passage. 'Like Ulysses' journey back home, you led us through Scylla and Charybdis as we heard the sirens tempting us in the distance,' explained a couple in their thank you card after a birth I attended some years ago.

Ringing the circle

The willing woman on the one hand wants to be held through a crisis of confidence, but on the other hand, when she's in the middle of a crisis, she wants to be let off the hook.

During a crisis of confidence, when the mother has lost her resolve to go on, she will begin searching the eyes of her support team. I've come to call this process of searching the eyes as 'ringing the circle'. What are they looking for? What will they find?

They're testing the circle. They are either looking for someone who will want to 'save' them and confirm that they can't do it—the 'weakest link'. Or, hopefully, they are looking for someone who can strengthen them—looking for their 'Dawn Fraser'.

If the mother is searching for the weakest link, searching for the way out, then her *partner* is often a fine way out: because out of his love and sympathy for her he is likely to crumble. The obstetrician, too, if they come in, will usually be a weak link, and the midwife might also be a weak link offering to make the mother comfortable.

Who will be your 'Dawn Fraser'? In terms of choosing a *support* team, you need to have people around who can hold solid for you, so that when you go searching their eyes, you don't see fear, you don't see pity, you don't see sympathy. You see someone mirroring your original aspiration, 'Yes, you can do it'.

Independent midwife Jennie says:

> Prior to the labour this has to be discussed. Why are you having this person here for you at this labour? Do you think they are really going to have faith in you and really trust? Is that person likely to worry and get distressed? Support people have to be carefully chosen.

Polly's story paints the picture.

> The pain was becoming unbearable—or at least, I had decided I wasn't strong enough to do it this time with my second baby. I looked around at my three support people, searching their eyes

for any hint of sympathy: an admission that what I was attempting was impossible and I could, therefore, give up now.

But no, their eyes betrayed no doubts, though my partner admitted afterwards that he had been filled with misery at my suffering this time. I zoomed in, pleadingly, on my midwife's eyes: she knew me least of the three, surely she would let me off. But her eyes gazed back, steadfast, confident.

Second stage was already harrowing but now I had to push as well. I felt myself beginning to lose it—I was drifting too far out now, getting lost in a big deep sea of pain. My team began calling me back, demanding I make eye contact. It was only through this focus that I was able to stay present enough to birth my big, beautiful baby girl.

The weakest link

Birthing women can become very creative in manoeuvring and working the team when these pain dynamics get going. Many will identify and target the 'weakest link' in their support circle. The birthing woman can usually smell the weakest link—the adrenalised smell of fear is a certain giveaway. If she can't *smell it*, she can certainly *see it*—in their eyes as she rings the circle. If she finds fear and sympathy in the same person then she knows she's hit the weakest-link jackpot!

If birthing women find a weak link, they will then often target them, as the following comment illustrates. In her story in *Birth Territory and Midwifery Guardianship*[87] Jane says:

> I confessed to my partner that I was really scared. I could see he was really anxious; he tried to be supportive but with each contraction I was saying 'I can't do it'. I chose him because, rather than make me face my fear, I knew he would agree with my beliefs that I couldn't do it …

It's a similar story in Michele's observations during her sister-in-law's labour:

> At its most intense, she was yelling and swearing at me. Meanwhile she was turning her back on me at regular intervals, desperately, but comparatively calmly, pleading with her partner to get a doctor because she couldn't cope with the pain. He looked so fearful and concerned and unsure—I remember it doing nothing for my confidence when my partner looked like this during our first baby's birth.

Birthing women seek the person who is pushed to their own limits of tiredness and exhaustion; or the person who does not hold, or have the experience to hold, a solid trust in either the birth process or the mother's capacity to accomplish it. Or they seek the person who, through fear, sympathy or lack of experience, will not be able to bear witnessing the demanding emotional and physical distress of a crisis of confidence.

Dena's story

Dena and Cameron's story illustrates a very creative 'weakest link' escape plan. They had invited me to join them for their first baby's birth at a birth centre. Dena explained that she wanted some extra support because she wasn't sure that she or Cameron would have the mental and emotional stamina demanded of them. Dena had given me the clear green light I required—permission to support her to keep to her intention of working with the normal functional pain of labour, even in the midst of a crisis of confidence. In this labour-bypass era, that green light was the leverage I needed in order to offer the intensity of support often required for normal physiological birth, especially in a first birth.

Even with this articulated between us before the labour, when it came to the reality, Dena was more challenged by the escalating intensity than she had imagined. Her self-doubts got going and she began to shape an elaborate plan to get herself out of 'the bloody support that I had set up!'

We'd been in phone contact overnight with early labour progressing well, but Dena could feel what the labour was going to ask of her and she didn't like it one bit! She could see that Cameron was also beginning to be worn down by the intensity. So her 'escape' plan was hatched. She felt she could work on Cameron's sympathy and she reckoned if she could get to the birth centre before I arrived, she was sure she could convince the midwives that she really did need that epidural. With this plan in mind she insisted on travelling to the birth centre during morning peak-hour traffic, knowing that it would take me longer to get there, by which time, as she told me later, 'the epidural would be a done deal!'

Luckily for the eventual outcome of her birth, but sadly for her escape plan, the traffic was not too heavy and I was able to get to the birth centre before she could complete her elaborate 'target the weakest link' plan.

The birth centre midwife met me and reported that Cameron had completely lost it. Dena was in a full-blown crisis and insisting that she transfer out of the birth centre for the epidural. The midwife said that stalling her was becoming very difficult, and that she hoped I could do something because the labour was going so beautifully and it would be a pity if Dena gave up now.

Usually, when I arrive at a birth, the birthing woman is pleased to see me. But not in Dena's case. She realised her escape plan was blown. During our time alone I was able to remind her that she had hit a crisis. I was able to connect with her enough to enable her to re-engage with her courage and intentions for the birth and find a way to surrender to her body's rhythm. She danced her way into the birth and some hours later met her sweet babe while squatting on a mat in the birth centre, just as she had originally intended.

The right support

When birthing women—even willing women, even women who in other areas of their life have a strong sense of personal agency, a can-do take on their world—are in a crisis of confidence and feeling that they can't do it, what then for the willing woman's intentions?

Who and what can fill the gap between her initial intentions and her now-crumbling self-belief and agency? This is where the facilitating holding circle comes in. First-time mother Natasha writes to a friend:

> Wowee. What a time I've been having. Giving birth was one of the most amazing experiences of my life! I had a girl in the lounge room at my mum and dad's house. I was open to having a water birth but the hot water had buggered up and the men (my father, brother and partner) were boiling pots of water to fill up the tub. It gave them a good excuse to leave the room. It's definitely women's work. The men felt very uncomfortable about seeing me 'in pain' and bellowing on all fours, but the women (my mother, sister, best friend and two midwives) were totally fine with it, even my sixteen-year-old sister.
>
> Finally she comes flying out and her dad caught her. Everyone is totally blown away. A special energy is in the room. I turned around with babe in arms to see my brothers, my mum and dad, my closest friend, my sister and midwives. Wowee, what a welcome!

So, willing woman: who will you choose to be with you to back your intentions for normal physiological birth? Who will offer the support you need so you can ride waves of confidence over any gaps in your own self-belief? Who will you choose to witness 'your show of strength' as midwife Jan describes it?

Birth support versus welcoming baby

Everyone I interviewed about working with pain, whether physical or psychological, pointed out that loved ones, partners or family are not automatically the best support for working with pain. Obviously loved ones provide much-needed love and nurture. However, at those confronting times in a sporting event, a play, writing a book or during a labour, when we are in crisis, loved ones may not be the people who can remain strong and guide us.

This truth is also supported by the latest research into continuous support in labour. After examining twenty-one trials involving over 15,000 women, the review authors for the *Cochrane Collaboration* found that: 'Continuous support from a person who is present solely to provide support, is not a member of the woman's social network, is experienced in providing labour support, and has at least a modest amount of training, appears to be most beneficial.'[88]

So, when thinking about who she will invite to be with her during the labour and birth of her baby, a willing woman needs to get clear about this distinction. Who are the experienced people she will need to aid her to work with the labour, as distinct from the people who will share the delight of welcoming her baby?

They may be the same people, but not necessarily. Many women don't take into account that both of these aspects—birth support and welcoming baby—call upon different qualities and therefore often need different people.

Obviously, welcoming the baby is a role for family and close friends, the people who will be involved in the ongoing life of your child, maybe the siblings of the coming baby, the grandparents, your sisters, brothers, aunts or friends. But these people may not be appropriate to support you through the hard work and functional pain of birthing. It's like relying on your personal trainer to get you through the marathon then embracing your family to celebrate at the finish line.

That's the difference between experienced support for the work of the achievement and the loving support for celebration of the achievement—or, in our case, for the welcome of the sweet, sweet baby.

Magic moments

Sometimes the support team needs to be as creative as the birthing woman to find some magic to hold the energy together.

Nature can often bring inspiration. I remember working with a woman having her first baby at home. She had reached a major crisis and was saying that she couldn't go on. Her entire birth team, partner, midwives and I had been using all our best expertise to work with her through this crisis, but she was still insisting that she couldn't go on, even though she understood that this meant she would have to transfer to hospital for pain relief.

All of the woman's and her baby's physical checks were strong, so that gave us some breathing space, but she was determined to go to the hospital. Just as this transfer seemed inevitable there came a magic moment.

I noticed that a harvest moon was coming up. The moon was very low on the horizon and looked absolutely huge and red. We turned the woman around until she was directly facing the moon, and she was captivated and inspired by it.

Talking about it with her later, she said it symbolised the life cycle for her and how, as human beings, we are pretty paltry in the scheme of those cycles. She felt that she could trust these cycles and so surrender to the forces of creation running through her body. This realisation meant she could let her ego-self dissolve and sink into trusting the cycles of change.

That moon was a gift. The circle held with its help. As the moon came up over the window ledge she started to push and as it rose to its zenith at the top of the window her baby boy was born.

Sometimes magic just happens. In dark, despairing moments, sometimes unexpected support appears that can change everything. Tammy van Wisse explains:

> It was a very bad stage of the Bass Strait swim. Apparently all my crew were thinking 'She's not going to make it, we're going to have to pull her out of the water', which was a shame because I think they could actually see Apollo Bay ten to fifteen kilometres away, not far. So here I am, I'm crying, I'm feeling so bad I'm wanting to vomit. I'm so cold. I was struggling. Luckily for me I had an outside influence.
>
> I got the message on the white board: 'We can see dolphins'. Well I love dolphins and it *totally* changed my focus and within

> a couple of minutes I had a pod of twenty dolphins swimming underneath the cage and the water is so crystal clear in the Bass that I could see down and there were actually a couple of babies, which is very unusual because normally when dolphins have young they don't come near humans. So I'm so excited. I turn around to Dawn and say stop the boat I'm getting out of the cage, I want to play with the dolphins.
>
> I hopped out of the cage and I had my couple of minutes of absolute euphoria with these dolphins that stayed and swam around me and did some somersaults underneath the water, and I guess I was on such a high after that, that I jumped back in the cage and the spirit and the feeling on board the boat from that moment on was that there was no way that I was not going to make it. You know afterwards they told me that some of them were crying. You know if you planned something like that you couldn't have done it at a better moment ... it was like they knew that I needed that particular lift at that stage. So it was two hours later and I landed at Apollo Bay and it was one of the greatest moments of my life.

Remember to always stay open to the possibility of magic. As Jo, mother of three, said after the birth of her last child:

> This was a truly emotional time and I found that although circumstances, environment and 'type of care' may change, there can always be that wonderful moment in birth that transcends all external influences. The challenge is to ensure this magical moment is not lost in all these influences, and that the true marvel of a new life joining us in this world is celebrated for its true wonder.

Before I leave you, I want to share with you one final story, one that shows how a willing woman, an 'oxytocinised' environment, knowledge and support can facilitate the normal process of birth and bonding.

Thaïs's story

During her second pregnancy and after a difficult first birth, Thaïs attended my weekly pregnancy sessions and invited me to be with her and her partner John for the birth.

> I ended up with an epidural, episiotomy and forceps for Will, my first baby. I'd pretty much covered it up and got on with life, as you do with a new baby, and I put up with a sore vagina, which meant I couldn't enjoy sex for a year after.
>
> I tried to debrief, talked to lots of people about the birth, wrote out my birth story … but it wasn't till I was pregnant with Ben that reality hit me. Going to Rhea's classes was like opening a Pandora's box: tears, fears, past, present. My second pregnancy with Ben was a journey of extreme emotion, working out and facing many fears.

After the birth of her second son Ben, Thaïs wrote him his birth story:

> When I went to bed that night it was only an hour before I felt deep waves beginning to rise up and around my pelvis and belly—they kept coming every six minutes.
>
> I went downstairs to wash some singlets and clothes to take with us to the Birth Centre—I knew you were on your way. I didn't tell anyone. I just wanted to do a normal day.
>
> It was about 6 pm when I stripped off my clothes and was rocking around the house. As each contraction started I'd sing into it and lean and rock and sway you. The music sucked away the pain. I was amazed how music that I knew well carried me through the contraction.
>
> John rang the birth centre and found out that my favourite midwife would be on duty—beauty. She hadn't arrived when we got there and my least favourite midwife was on. I knew I had to make it work so that I could birth you. With the next contraction I held that midwife and asked her for a huge hug—something

shifted, we were able to go on. Rhea arrived, she and the midwife knew each other and it made the energy easy and smooth.

'I don't think I can do this anymore', I said to Rhea. 'How much longer?' 'Best not to think about it,' she said. 'Just take it moment by moment.' We put on my music and I hung from the big silk swathe of material hanging from the ceiling

It fucking killed! I was totally deep inside and silent. Rhea honoured my pain as I went into each contraction, just requesting the others be silent with me till it passed. I needed to know everyone was there with me supporting me one hundred percent.

Suddenly the silence turned to *roar, groan, push!* I had my head down watching the hot water splash in drops. It was running hot on my back but I was panicking. I still felt a contraction working on my cervix but also the urge to push. Help! The memory of the same premature urge to push flashed back from Will's birth. Rhea knew. She just said 'Can you still feel more cervix to come up in the front?' I could. She crouched down with her head on the wet tiles … I needed her to be totally with me as we 'ah, ah, oohed'.

I'd heard many people talk about focussing on someone's eyes during labour. When I had the urge to push but still had some cervix to come up I had to focus on Rhea's eyes and mouth and breathe and pant.

Then I knew you were ready to come out. I looked up and saw my favourite midwife had arrived—bliss! I totally trusted her and I totally trusted Rhea that it was now okay and safe to go into the push. Johno was there, the other midwife was with us; such a beautiful supportive team. I trusted them to honour my strength and be totally rigorous if need be, and not give into me! It was perfect.

I moved into the warm room shaking and supported on each side. I was burning down the outside of my pelvis—fuck it killed! I felt so shaky and weak … yet I knew I was about to do the most powerful thing ever in my life.

> It took about an hour to push you out but it felt like five minutes and eternity at the same time: Help! Fuck! Fuck! How am I going to push you out that tiny hole? How the fuck is my fanny going to stretch that far?
>
> 'You're going to push this baby out with the next push,' said Rhea, but I didn't for the next two pushes. Talking to Rhea I realised I didn't want to let you go to be snatched up by everyone like Will was. I wanted to let you go and share you with others at the right time for you and me. Once [I said it], it was okay; I wished you a wonderful life and then with the next push John caught your head; then your body slipped out. So, so, so beautiful—I was just silent and we sat quietly with you for a long while.

Thaïs reflected later on the birth:

> I was blown away by the things that helped me to birth Ben naturally. The team who all knew one another really well and, together with John, created such a peaceful, strong, rigorous and loving support circle. And I wonder how different Will's birth may have been if I'd had access to the same support and knowledge.

Conclusion

My hope is that after reading this book, willing women, you, like Thaïs, are able to bring together all the elements—the savvy choices and birthing wisdom—that can give you the best opportunity for a normal physiological birth to unfold.

I hope I have given you an awareness of the challenges and obstacles you face in undertaking such a birth in our labour-bypass era, that you can see the impact of our current lifestyle on your birthing capacity and are able to reframe your attitude to pain in labour. I hope that you will make intelligent, informed choices about the best support people to see you through any crisis of confidence in labour.

I hope that, in reading this book and making savvy choices, you can avoid the kind of experience I had during my first daughter's birth all those years ago, and instead labour in a beautifully 'oxytocinised' space with the right support to enable you to birth with power, courage and confidence. It is my heartfelt hope that you are able to birth normally, as you desire, so that your baby can emerge, into that 'love bomb' of hormones—showering benefits on you, your baby, your partner and all the loved ones gathered around to receive your new baby into their hearts.

Personal reflection

- So are you a willing woman—a savvy willing woman?
- Have you made the wise choices that will support you to achieve a normal physiological birth?
- Are you in touch with your instincts and will you be able to surrender to your birth dance and song?
- Will you be able to normalise any crisis of confidence moments?
- Who is supporting you at the birth?
- What are you basing your birth support choices on?
- Have you got a facilitating team around you?
- Have you experienced the support of a facilitating environment—a facilitating holding circle—in any area of achievement in your life?
- Will you be able to apply that experience to the birth of your baby?
- Are you ready to approach the challenge of birthing; ready to be supported into your strength; ready to surrender to the mystery of transformation and ready to bond deeply with your baby while luxuriating in that oxytocin lurve haze?

Further reading

Balaskas, J. (1989) *New Active Birth.* United Kingdom.

Balaskas, J. (1992) *Water Birth: the conscise guide to using water during pregnancy, birth and infancy*. United Kingdom: Woolnough Bookbinding Ltd.

Beech, B. (2003) *Am I Allowed?* United Kingdom: AIMS (Association for Improvements in the Maternity Services).

Buckley, S. (2012) *Gentle Birth Gentle Mothering: a doctors guide to natural childbirth and parenting choices.* United States: Celestial Arts.

Davis-Floyd, R. (1992) *Birth as an American Rite of Passage.* California: University of California Press.

Davis-Floyd, R. and Sargeant, C. (1997) *Childbirth and Authoritative knowledge: cross cultural perspectives.* California, United States: University of California Press.

Goer, H. (1999) *The Thinking Woman's Guide to a Better Birth.* New York, United States: Berkley Publishing Group.

Kitzinger, S. (2006) *Birth Crisis.* United Kingdom: Routlege.

Kitzinger, S. (2005) *The Politics of Birth.* United Kingdom: Elsevier Ltd.

Kitzinger, S. (2010) *The New Pregnancy and Childbirth.* United Kingdom.

MacColl, M. (2009) *The Birth Wars.* Queensland, Australia: University of Queensland Press.

Sundin, J. (2007) *Birth Skills.* Australia: Allen and Unwin.

Wickham, S. (2002) *Making Decisions in Pregnancy and Birth.* United Kingdom: AIMS (Association for Improvements in the Maternity Services).

References

Chapter 1

1 Lopez, S. and Snyder, C. (2009) *Oxford Handbook of Positive Psychology.* United States: Oxford University Press.

2 Seligman, M. (2011) *Flourish: a visionary new understanding of happiness and well-being.* United States: Free Press.

3 Hooton, A. (2012) 'All Psyched Up'. *The Age*, 11 July 2012.

4 Dallenbach, R. et al. (2012) *Sustainability, Midwifery and Birth.* England.

5 Gibbons, L. et al. (2010) 'The Global Numbers and Costs of Additionally Needed and Unnecessary Caesarean Sections Performed Per Year: overuse as a barrier to universal coverage'. World Health Organisation, no. 30 (Background Paper).

6 Marshall, H. et al. (2002) *The Doula Book: how a trained labour companion can help you have a shorter, easier and healthier birth.* 2nd ed. United States: Perseus Publishing.

7 Alfirevic, Z. et al. (2009) *A Cochrane Pocketbook of Pregnancy & Childbirth.* Sussex, United Kingdom: John Wiley & Sons.

8 Page, LA. (ed) (2000) *The New Midwifery: science and sensitivity in practice.* Edinburgh, United Kingdom: Churchill Livingston.

9 McLachlan, HL. et al. (2012) 'Effects of Continuity of Care by Primary Midwife (Caseload Midwifery) on Caesarean Section Rates in Women of Low Obstetric Risk: the COSMOS randomized controlled trial'. *British Journal of Obstetrics and Gynaecology An International Journal of Obstetrics and Gynaecology.*

10 Medew, J. (2012) 'Dedicated Midwives a Boon to Births: study'. *The Age*, 26 July 2012.

11 Guililand, K. and Pairman, S. (1995) *The Midwifery Partnership: a model for practice.* Wellington, New Zealand: Department of Nursing and Midwifery, Victoria University.

12 Fahy, K. et al. (2008) *Birth Territory and Midwifery Guardianship.* United Kingdom: Elsevier Ltd.

13 Dahlen, H. (2011) 'Home Births: it's time to broaden the focus of the debate'. Crikey.com.au, [online] 14 November 2011. Available at: www.crikey.com.au [Accessed: 15 November 2011].
14 Kotaska, A. 'Guideline-Centered Care: a two-edged sword.' *Birth Issues in Perinatal Care*. June 2011 (38:2).
15 Mander, R. (2011) 'They're only words ...'. MIDIRS Midwifery Digest, 21 (4).

Chapter 2

16 Dahlen, H. (2011) 'Home Births: it's time to broaden the focus of the debate'. loc. cit.
17 World Health Organization (WHO) Fortelesa Declaration (1985) 'Appropriate technology for birth'. *Lancet*, 2. 24 August 1985, pp 436–437.
18 Eldridge, D. et al. (2016) Australia's Mothers and Babies 2014 Australian Institute of Health and Welfare, Perinatal statistics series no. 32.
19 ibid.
20 Davey, M. (2012) 'Private Hospital Births: "horror" figures'. *The Age*, 10 September 2012.
21 Dahlen, H. et al. (2012) 'Rates of Obstetric Intervention Among Low-Risk Women Giving Birth in Private and Public Hospitals in NSW: a population-based descriptive study'. *British Medical Journal Open*.
22 Horsley, E. (2012) 'On Beyond Cambridge: a journey of healing through continuity of care'. *Birth Matters: journal of Maternity Coalition,* 16 (2), pp 12–13.
23 Chalmers, I. et al. (2012) *Effective Care in Pregnancy and Childbirth.* United States: Oxford University Press.
24 Wallace, E. (2011) *The Face of Birth* [dvd]. Australia: Kate Gorman.
25 LaFortune, G. et al. (2011) 'Health at a Glance: OECD indicators'. *OECD*, http://www.oecd.org/dataoecd/6/28/49105858.pdf.9.
26 Powell Kennedy, H. et al. (2010) 'Normalising Birth in England: a qualitative study'. *Midwifery Women's Health*, 55 (3), pp 262–269.
27 Royal College of Midwives. (2007) 'Making Normal Birth a Reality: consensus statement from the Maternity Care Working Party' [press release]. November 2007.

28 Gourounti, K. and Sandall, J. (2007) 'Intrapartum Admission Cadiotocography (CTG) Versus Intermittent Auscultation of Fetal Heart Rate: a meta-analysis'. *International Journal of Nursing Studies.*,44 (6), pp 1029–1035.

29 De Vries, R. (2004) *A Pleasing Birth: midwives and maternity care in the Netherlands.* Philadelphia, United States: Temple University Press.

30 Groopman, J. and Hartzband, P. (2012) *Your Medical Choices: how to decide what is right for you. Australia*: Scribe.

31 Thaler, R. and Sunstein, C. (2008) *Nudge: improving decisions about health, wealth and happiness.* United States: Yale University Press.

32 LaFortune, G. et al. (2011) 'Health at a Glance: OECD indicators'. *OECD*. loc. cit.

33 Howell, C. et al. (2009) 'Epidural Versus Non-Epidural for Pain Relief in Labour'. *A Cochrane Pocketbook of Pregnancy & Childbirth.* Sussex, United Kingdom: John Wiley & Sons.

34 Moberg, K. (2003) *The Oxytocin Factor: tapping the hormone of calm, love and healing.* United States: Da Capo Press.

35 Odent, M. (2004) *The Caesarean.* United Kingdom: Free Association Books.

Chapter 3

36 Williams, J. (1988) *Applied Sport Psychology: personal growth to peak performance.* 3rd ed. California, United States: Mayfield Publishing Company.

37 Stark, J. (2009) 'Doctors Warn of New Drug Crisis as Painkiller-Pill Addiction Soars'. *The Sunday Age*, 27 September 2009.

38 Mongan, M. (2005) *Hypnobirthing: the mongan method: a natural approach to a safe, easier more comfortable birthing.* 3rd ed. Florida, United States: Health Communications.

39 Davis, E. and Pascali-Bonaro, D. (2010) *Orgasmic Birth: your guide to a safe, satisfying and pleasurable birth experience.* United States: Rodale Inc.

40 Dempsey, R. (1997) 'Pain is Power'. Women & Labour Conference proceedings: Deakin University Geelong. December 1997.

41 Moberg, K. (2003) *The Oxytocin Factor: tapping the hormone of calm, love and healing.* loc. cit.

42 Gaskin, I. (2003) *Ina May's Guide to Childbirth.* New York, United States: Bantam Dell.

43 Dowrick, S. (2012) *The Universal Heart: golden rules for golden relationships.* Australia: Penguin Books.

44 Szalavitz, M. and Perry, B. (2010) *Born for Love: why empathy is essential – and endangered.* New York, United States: HarperCollins.

45 Powell Kennedy, H. et al. (2010) 'Normalising Birth in England: a qualitative study'. *Midwifery Women's Health*, 55 (3), pp 262–269.

46 Fahy, K. et al. (2008) *Birth Territory and Midwifery Guardianship.* loc. cit.

47 Davies, L. (2007) *The Art and Soul of Midwifery: creativity in practice.* United States: Elsevier Ltd.

Chapter 4

48 Reiger, K. and Dempsey, R. (2006) 'Performing Birth in a Culture of Fear: an embodied crisis of late modernity'. *Health Sociology Review*, 15 (4).

49 Fahy, K. et al. (2008) *Birth Territory and Midwifery Guardianship.* loc. cit.

50 Leap, N. (1998) 'A Fresh Approach to Pain in Labour'. *New Zealand College of Midwives Journal*, 19, pp 17–18.

51 Leap, N. (2000) 'Pain in labour'. *MIDIRS Midwifery Digest*, 10 (1), pp 49–53.

52 Leap, N. et al. (2010) 'Working With Pain in Labour: an overview of evidence'. *New Digest*, January, pp 22–26.

53 Horsley, E. (2012) 'On Beyond Cambridge: a journey of healing through continuity of care'. loc. cit.

54 Mander, R. (2011) *Pain in Childbearing and its Control.* 2nd ed. West Sussex, United Kingdom: John Wiley & Sons Ltd.

55 Dahlen, H. (2011) 'Home Births: it's time to broaden the focus of the debate'. loc. cit.

Chapter 5

56 Morey, P. (1999) 'Sighed, Squealed and Delivered'. *The Weekend Australian*, 13 February 1999.

57 Dempsey, R. (1996) 'The Emotional Journey of Labour: birth of a mother'. Birth Issues Conference proceedings. 28 November–1 December, pp 55–61.

58 Dempsey, R. (1998) 'Embracing the Intensity: celebrating birth as a peak bodily performance'. National Conference of National Association of Childbirth Educators. Melbourne. 15–17 August 1998.

59 Guppy, J. (2011) 'Baring It All for Art'. Interviewed by Jeanavive McGregor. Australia: Radio National.

60 Dempsey, R. (2001) 'Embracing the Intensity Part II: celebrating birth as a challenging life process'. National Conference of National Association of Childbirth Educators. Brisbane. 27–29 April 2001.

61 Mc Girr, M. (2011) 'The Passion of Arts Seduction'. *The Age*, 15 October 2011.

62 The Age Good Weekend Magazine (2009). Interview with Jane Campion on the making of *Bright Star.* 5 December 2009.

63 Dempsey, R. (2001) 'Embracing the Intensity Part II: celebrating birth as a challenging life process'. loc. cit.

64 ibid.

65 Morey, P. (1999) 'Sighed, Squealed and Delivered'. loc. cit.

66 Dempsey, R. (2001) Embracing the Intensity Part II: celebrating birth as a challenging life process'. loc. cit.

67 Hartley, L. (1995) *Wisdom of the Body Moving: an introduction to body-mind centering.* California, United States: North Atlantic Books.

68 Gendlin, E. (1996) *Focusing-Oriented Psychotherapy: a manual of the experiential method.* New York, United States: Guilford Press.

69 De Braganca, M. and Sposato, N. (2010) Strange Fruit performers. Interviewed by Rhea Dempsey [in person]. Melbourne, Australia, 15 May 2010.

70 Dempsey, R. (2010) 'Playing with Wildcards'. *National Conference of* National Association of Childbirth Educators. Brisbane.

71 Dempsey, R. (2011) 'Post Traumatic Stress Disorder Resulting from Childbirth'. *Maternal and Child Health Newsletter.* Melbourne. February 2011.

72 Horsley, E. (2012) 'On Beyond Cambridge: a journey of healing through continuity of care'. *loc. cit.*

Chapter 6

73 Dempsey, R. (2001) 'Embracing the Intensity Part II: celebrating birth as a challenging life process'. loc. cit.

74 De Braganca, M. and Sposato, N. (2010) Strange Fruit performers. loc. cit.

75 ibid.

76 Dempsey, R. (2001) 'Embracing the Intensity part II: celebrating birth as a challenging life process'. loc. cit.

77 ibid.

78 Winnicott, D. (1992) *Babies and their Mothers.* Massachusetts, United States: Addison-Wesley Publishing Company.

79 Dempsey, R. (2001) 'Embracing the Intensity Part II: celebrating birth as a challenging life process'. loc. cit.

80 ibid.

81 Siegel, A. (1996) *Heinz Kohut and the Psychology of the Self.* United States: Routledge.

82 Dempsey, R. (2001) 'Embracing the Intensity Part II: celebrating birth as a challenging life process'. loc. cit.

83 Vincent, A. (2011) Untitled. *Dad's Blog* [online]. Available at: www.adamvincent.com [Accessed: 17 June 2012].

84 Dempsey, R. (2001) 'Embracing the Intensity Part II: celebrating birth as a challenging life process'. loc. cit.

85 Groopman, J. and Hartzband, P. (2012) *Your Medical Choices: how to decide what is right for you*. loc. cit.

86 Thaler, R. and Sunstein, C. (2008) *Nudge: improving decisions about health, wealth and happiness*. loc. cit.

87 Fahy, K. et al. (2008) *Birth Territory and Midwifery Guardianship.* loc. cit.

88 Alfirevic, Z. et al. (2009) *A Cochrane Pocketbook of Pregnancy & Childbirth.* loc. cit.

Acknowledgements

Thank you to my mother who birthed me and, with my father, loved my siblings and me enough to create a warm and loving extended family. Thank you to both my parents and my siblings, particularly my sister Liz, for supporting my work and the long gestation of this book.

Thank you to Trevor, the father of my daughters, who was beside me through their births and growing years. Thank you to my daughters who, through their births, awakened and deepened my interest in birth. Thank you for each offering your unique richness to my life. Matthia, who awakened me as a mother and stirred my passion for birth work. Darcy, who awakened my trust and delight in birthing. Sonia, who awakened my awareness that each baby has its own timing, nature and purpose.

Thank you to the editors: Megan for her timely encouragement and overview, Jo for the line edit, Irma for the fresh eyes and, most importantly, my daughter Matthia, who has not only awakened my life's work but has also, through her role as my editor, offered warmth, attention to detail, skill, belief in my words and fortitude during many crises of confidence. She has guided and expertly shaped this distilling of the insights gained from my years of birth work.

Thank you to the early transcribers of interviews, Fleur and Erica, and more recent typists, especially my daughter Sonia, who struggled through my handwriting and disjointed musings. Thank you Leigh, for braving the end notes and so much more, also Milly, Narelle and Sonia for administrative support.

Thank you to the early readers: Irma, Melinda, Chris, Melissa, Jess, Halimah, Alexandra, Kay and Tim; and, more recently, Michelle, Sophie, Justine, Maria, Kerreen, Jennie, Shantah and Leigh. Thank you for your valuable feedback across the various versions that finally culminated in this finished book.

Thank you also to Sue, Shantah, Eugenia and Andrew for the needed writing retreats.

Thank you to the designers Megan, Sandra, Keith and Latifah for the to-the-point, pared back simple elegance of the book, which is (I hope) in keeping with the content. And thank you to Cinzia for her publishing knowledge and advice.

Thank you to the athletes, swimmers, dancers, circus and physical performers, writers, actors and directors who agreed to speak with me about crisis of confidence experiences in their own activities. Thank you also to Anna and others for the philosophical discussions about 'birth' as a portal into everything.

Thank you to my early mentors in birth work—Jan, Mel and Maree. Also, vale Bettye; I miss your gentle presence. Thank you to the many midwives, childbirth educators, birth attendants and birth activists who have shared their knowledge and their passion for birth, mothers, babies and families with me.

Thank you to those at the organisations—the Childbirth and Parenting Educators of Australia (CAPEA), Maternity Coalition (MC) and Choices for Childbirth—for the work you do and for the continued support and encouragement of my work.

Finally, thank you to all the birthing women, partners and sweet babies, for inviting me to share your intimate birth moments; for the generosity; for the stories, both those shared here and the many more that have added richness to my understanding. Thank you for the stories of delight and the stories of courage in the face of despair. I trust I have done them justice.

I also trust that this distilling of years of involvement in birth work is useful for willing women and all the babies to come.

Rhea
Melbourne 2013
www.birthingwisdom.com.au